The Unfashionable Human Body

The Unfashionable Human Body

Bernard Rudofsky

VNR VAN NOSTRAND REINHOLD COMPANY
New York

Copyright © 1971 by Bernard Rudofsky
Copyright 1947 by Paul Theobold
Library of Congress Catalog Card Number 84-17429

ISBN 0-442-27636-2

Printed in the United States of America
Designed by Bernard Rudofsky

The chapter "The fashionable body" and part of "Anatomy of modesty"
first appeared in *Horizon* magazine.

Published in 1984 by Van Nostrand Reinhold Company Inc.
135 West 50th Street
New York, New York 10020

Van Nostrand Reinhold Company Limited
Molly Millars Lane
Wokingham, Berkshire RG11 2PY, England

Van Nostrand Reinhold
480 La Trobe Street
Melbourne, Victoria 3000, Australia

Macmillan of Canada
Division of Gage Publishing Limited
164 Commander Boulevard
Agincourt, Ontario M1S 3C7, Canada

First published by Doubleday & Company, Inc.

16   15   14   13   12   11   10   9   8   7   6   5   4   3   2   1

Library of Congress Cataloging in Publication Data

Rudofsky, Bernard, 1905–
    The unfashionable human body.

    Reprint. Originally published: Garden City, N.Y.:
Doubleday, 1971.
    Bibliography: p.
    Includes index.
    1. Costume—History.   2. Nudity.   3. Human figure in
art. I. Title.
GT510.R76   1984   391   84-17429
ISBN 0-442-27636-2

Contents

Acknowledgements

I wish to acknowledge old and current debts of gratitude to my editor, Anne Freedgood. I am greatly obliged to the editors of *Horizon* for permission to include a chapter published in their magazine; to the editors of *Vogue* for furnishing me a number of excellent photographs, and to the staff of the Photothèque at the Musée de l'Homme in Paris. Special thanks go to Saul Steinberg for doing a face painting expressly for this book, and granting me the use of three drawings, and to Bernard Pfriem who accomplished the painterly feat of overreaching human anatomy. I am much indebted to Eliot Elisofon for his generosity in availing me pictures from his archive; to William Klein and the ineffable Christo for supplying photographs of their work. I also want to extend my thanks to Andrea Womack, Sigrid Spaeth, and Lisa Guerrero for graciously giving their time to modeling. As always, the greatest tribute goes to my wife, constant helper and sincerest critic. Parts of this book are based on my 1944 exhibition "Are Clothes Modern?" at the Museum of Modern Art in New York, and my book of the same title.

Foreword

Next morning the prince went to his father, the King, and said to him: "No one shall be my wife but she whose foot this golden slipper fits." Then were the two sisters glad, for they had pretty feet. The eldest went with the shoe into her room and wanted to try it on, and her mother stood by. But she could not get her big toe into it, and the shoe was too small for her. Then her mother gave her a knife and said: "Cut the toe off, when thou art Queen thou wilt no more need to go on foot." The maiden cut the toe off, forced the foot into the shoe, swallowed the pain, and went out to the King's son. Then he took her on his horse as his bride and rode away with her.[1]

He was, alas, not an observant man. He galloped away with barely a glance at his prey; she might have been lame, for all he cared. But this was not the happy end; the Grimms' story continues with the discovery of the fraud. Blood, streaming from the bride's shoe, has dyed her white stockings red, making a mess and crowding the symbols. Calling the bluff, the prince returns the misfit whereupon the mother, undaunted, fobs off her second daughter on the gullible bridegroom—not without first having shrunk her foot by amputating its heel. Again, the deceit is bloodily revealed, and the prince returns the wrong bride. This time he meets Cinderella. Virtue, equated by shoe size, triumphs when the prince finds the foot of his dreams.

The tale of Cinderella, a veritable case history from the psychopathology of dress, has its protagonists made to order for the couch: The august shoe fetishist who turns the country upside down to satisfy his craving for a miniature foot; the maniacal mother with the instincts of a procuress and the tenderness of a hangman; and the unappreciated heroines of the story—obedient daughters and true martyrs in the cause of sartorial perfection—whose keepsakes from the sleaziest of all love affairs are mangled feet. Only Cinderella, the serene dummy, emerges untouched by problems and passions.

At bedtime, this tale is whispered to eager ears to linger forever in children's memories. At a tender age, even before they can distinguish between good and evil, they learn of the magic power of dress—how love and security await the good girl who unreservedly complies with the tastes of man.

American children are spared the gory details of the original story by being fed a vegetarian, pumpkin-coach version of Cinderella. In the eighteen-nineties, the heyday of gentility, the mother's scheming and ensuing surgery fell victim to the censor. The blood-soaked shoes were replaced by aseptic glass slippers. A Boston edition of the Grimms' *Tales* omits Cinderella altogether. Its foreword states with stern satisfaction: " . . . when the objectionable stories have been thrown out, there remains a goodly number."[2]

Yet even the numberless bowdlerized versions of Cinderella cannot fail to impress children with the fact that the choice of the sovereign princess depended on her shoe size. Curiously, the fascination with disproportionately small feet is not just the outcrop of a scabrous mind but stems from the belief that a tiny foot goes with a small vagina. Although the original association has been palliated, if not altogether forgotten, the bias in favor of infant-size female feet remains intact. For ages women have squeezed their feet into shoes that were far too small for them, blessedly unaware of the implications. "The smallness of the foot," wrote a French physician living in Pékin in the middle of the last century, "is not the criterion

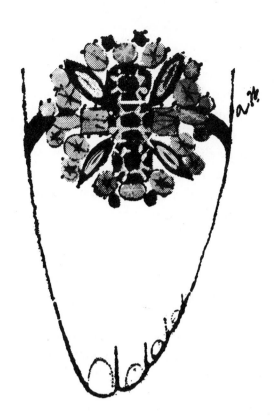

Drawing by Andy Warhol
for an advertisement. 1952.
(Courtesy, I. Miller Shoes)

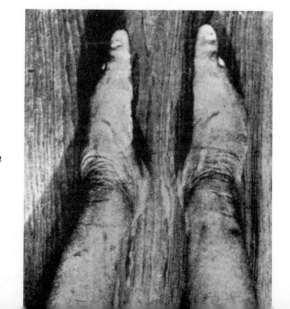

Correctly shaped feet of a Chinese woman
from the time before the revolution.

of her beauty, but of a woman's commercial value. The bride's shoe is exhibited before the bridegroom's parents and figures as one of the deciding arguments in determining the price of purchase."[3] In the China of old, dwarfing a woman's feet—which was accomplished by dislocating their bones—was believed to produce hypertrophy of her sexual parts. The Chinese, our informant speculated, applied experience gained from horticulture, where certain branches are sacrificed in order to feed others. The disfigurement of the toes, though repulsive, was of no concern to them. Among shoe-wearing peoples, men are perfectly content to take the shoe for the foot.

Usually, we let matters rest there without feeling displeased with ourselves; we concede to apparel and its encroachments on our anatomy an illogicalness all their own. Dress, we have decided, though often absurd, produces delights that outweigh discomfort and organic disorders. All our attempts to overcome this obsession by rationalizing the nature of dress have failed. The utilitarian sees in dress no more than a protection from the elements, although the example of races who brave the rigors of a cold climate without benefit of clothes tends to discredit this belief. Equally untenable is the argument that the habit of wearing clothes is due to modesty. We have to remember that many naked tribes put on clothes only for dances whose object it is to excite the passion of the opposite sex. Still another theory attributes the origin of dress to man's love of ornament. Yet ornament does not help to protect or conceal the body. Quite the contrary; it emphasizes its nakedness.

Be that as it may, I cannot pass over these contradictory opinions without airing my own thoughts on the nature of apparel. It seems that man's and animals' clothes serve much the same purpose—sexual selection. Only the roles of the sexes are reversed. In the animal kindgom it is the male who infatuates the female with his gorgeous garb. She falls for his looks rather than his strength and aggressiveness. In human society on the other hand, the burden is on the woman. Hers is the first move; she has to track and ensnare the male by looking seductive. Being devoid of anything comparable to the extraordinary antennae and giant legs that serve animals for prehending a partner, she exerts her powers by way of artificial plumage. To prevent the male from escaping, she has to keep him perpetually excited by changing her shape and colors by every means, fair and foul. In the traditional battle of the sexes, dress and its accessory arts are her offensive weapons.

Whichever way we look at clothes, one factor stands out—our inability, or unwillingness, to settle for a type of dress of more than passing interest. Our dissatisfaction with the body and its coverings expresses itself in ceaseless change. Each new dress becomes something like an accomplice with whom we enter a most intimate, if brief, relationship. The first stirrings of timid desire for the adoption of a fad; the intense devotion to it while it lasts; the sudden boredom and physical revulsion for an outlived vogue—all these are the perfect analogy to the phases of courtship: craving for the love object, and its rejection after wish fulfillment. When the excitement over a new fashion flares up, symbols of old come miraculously alive; strange cruelties and mutilations are accepted in homage of an idol that, were its nature fully understood, would scare the wits out of its adherents.

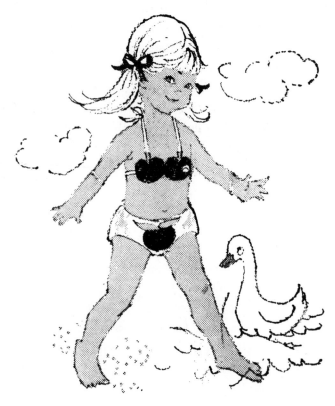

a saucy bikini for the apple of your eye! **3.98**

The child's outfit illustrates, as it were, a quaint version of the Fall according to which the halves of the fateful apple, or apples, were grafted on to the sinners in the form of breasts and testicles. In antiquity the apple symbolized love; offering an apple to one's inamorata—a gesture familiar to us from the Judgment of Paris— equaled a declaration of love. Later, the apple became a symbol of seduction and mischief, perhaps because in Latin malum *means both, apple and evil.*
(Courtesy, Arnold Constable)

The birth of clothes

Man which glories in his raiment
is like a robber that glories in the
brand of irons wherewith he is
branded, since it was Adam's sin
that rendered garments necessary.

St. Bernard

In an unauthorized easterly version of the Fall, the first man and woman are described as sexless; only after having sinned "were the halves of the forbidden apple grafted unto them in the shape of breasts and testicles." This interpretation would seem preferable to that of the Bible—if only for its poetic imagery—were it not that it leaves one puzzled in more than one respect. While it illuminates in an oblique way the disenchantment that had befallen Creation, it sheds no light on the protagonists' physical condition *before* the Fall. For what could be more awkward than the thought of a dalliance between sexually void ancestors—two bungled creatures instead of healthy working models of humanity. The parable is not exactly edifying; although it helps to pinpoint the seats of shame, it does not hint at the downright insurmountable difficulties faced by a sexless couple bent on sinning. Moreover, the story contains a baffling piece of intelligence which to this day prevents us from forming an unbiased view of the human body—the definition of our sexual organs as badges of sin. Still, one is bound to admire the Lord's resourcefulness; rather than, say, cutting off the sinners' noses or ears, he tagged them, as it were, with appendages that henceforth are identified with shame.

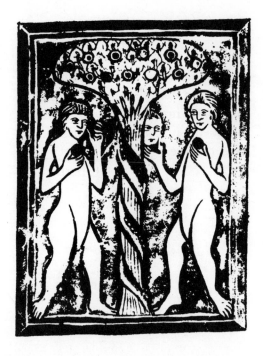

Which one is Adam, which one is Eve? The fourteenth-century woodcut shows a sexless couple on the point of sinning, with their innocence and their apples still intact..

An equally haunting account of the Fall, a tale from, of all places, Nepal, vigorously contradicts the foregoing. It credits the original humans with being androgynous, conferring upon them the doubtful privilege of being equipped with the characteristics of *both* sexes. Again, this attribution poses a question: How was the embarrassment of riches resolved for the benefit of posterity? Since Adam and Eve had no way of *disguising* themselves as man and woman —clothes had yet to be invented—how did they differ from each other? Which one was Adam, which one was Eve?

Despite its remote origin, the story does not sound unfamiliar, for it echoes Talmudic doctrine where primitive humanity is bisexual. Moreover, it not only tallies with Arabic esotericism, it also agrees with Aristophanes' view on the beginnings of the human race that he expressed in Plato's *Symposium*. In Aristophanes' opinion the earliest human beings did not belong to either sex but had double organs; "they were man and woman at the same time."

These sensuous fabrications of folklore and mythology, bristling with subtleties and indiscretions, suggest that by relying exclusively on the account of the Fall as told in the Scriptures we are depriving ourselves of a good deal of spiritual uplift. To make some headway into the shrouded past, we must turn to theological casuistry. One ponderer who was particularly successful in unraveling the knotty circumstances that obscure the nature of the first man is the eighteenth-century mystic Jacob Boehme. Harking back to Aristophanes, he spun out his allegories of primeval Adam in colorful language, adding archaic nuances as he went along. "Adam," he argued, "was a man and also a woman, and yet none of them, but a virgin full of chastity, modesty, and purity, viz., the image of God."[4] His Adam emerges as a semi-divine, albeit fumbling creature, a near equal of the angels whose sex, if any, has likewise remained a matter of speculation. He walked naked upon the earth, and could do so with impunity, Boehme assures us, because "the

17

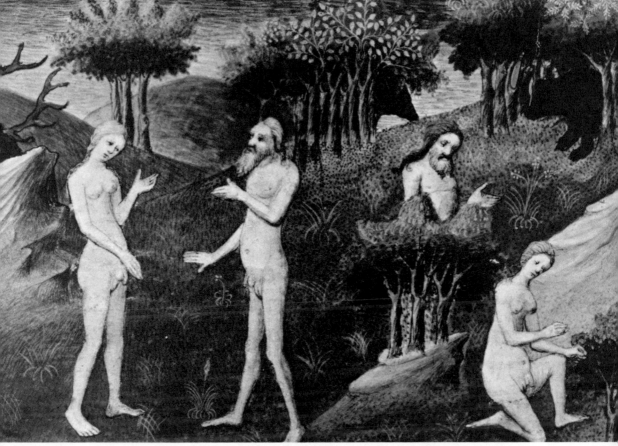

In this thirteenth-century miniature, Adam and Eve are portrayed in their early paradisiacal splendor, both equipped with male and female genitals. (Courtesy, Bibliothèque Nationale, Paris)

heavenly part [his angelesque inner constitution] penetrated the outward, *and was his clothing*."[5] This garment, a sort of supernatural oxygen tent, which also turns up in the two following episodes, probably was akin in appearance to the halos and halo-leotards of the saints. At any rate, it was a clever device for clothing the naked without looking nudity in the eye.

If Boehme's argument strikes us as a trifle vaporous, he subsequently endears himself to us with his unanswerable logic: "If God had created Adam to the earthly, toilsome life, then He had not brought him into Paradise; if He had desired, or willed, the bestial copulation and propagation, He then would instantly in the beginning have created man and woman . . . "[6] In other words, He would have fitted man and woman all along with their respective sexual parts.

To give American theologians their due—a contemporary of Boehme's, one Charles Chauncey, minister of the Fifth Church in Boston, the author of five dissertations on the Scriptures' account of the Fall, went one step further by maintaining that innocence and nakedness are incompatible. That may very well have been true for his parish but to make his point he felt it his duty to improve on chapter three of Genesis by covering up the as yet untested First Parents with "robes of glory," a kind of metaphysical négligé. The overfastidious Chauncey, who had what William James called the perfect pitch of New England sensibility, simply could not bring himself to admit the thought of the fallen pair clad in anything as flimsy as theology's fig leaves. Such a half-measure was unacceptable to him; as he put it, only by "casing themselves up with boughs full of leaves, to look like trees,"[7]—hence the expression full fig—did they become presentable to the eyes of God. (We shall return to the provisional fig-leaf costumes in a moment.) It did not occur to Chauncey that the Lord, being omniscient, could see perfectly well through the camouflage. Yet the extra precautions attributed to Adam no doubt satisfied his audience.

It also was Chauncey's idea to have Adam borrow his earlier "robe of light" from the Lord's own wardrobe (Psalm 104:2, "Who coverest Thyself with *light* as with a garment"). The use of such a garment was quite common among Olympians. Beclouded, star-spangled clothes seem to have been regular outfits of such dissimilar deities as the Canaanite Baal, the Teutonic Odin, and the African Maiou. Even one Jewish legend—every bit as ingenious and ambiguous as the above-mentioned ones—concurs with Reverend Chauncey in not allowing an innocent *naked* Adam. "A horny skin," so it says, "covered his body, and *the Lord's cloud surrounded him at all times*. But after he ate from the fruits of the tree, his horny skin was wrested from him and the cloud melted away. He looked at his nakedness and hid from the Lord."[8] (Italics added.)

This picture of the fallen Adam as a kind of peeled shrimp is no more fanciful than our own Bible version. What seem to us quaint speculations are, however, hard facts to the child who gets his basic orientation in Sunday school where modesty, a virtue both complex and irrational, is implanted in his mind by means of equally complex and irrational allegories. Instead of underpinning his faith in man, we give him moral goose-pimples. Far from mending the breach between mind and body, we try to repair the irreparable by bundling him into clothes; by ramming him down, as it were, into an esoteric, secondhand shell. The shell cracks alternatingly or simultaneously in several places, sometimes to the unconcealed delight of its wearer. And although the observance of the dictates of modesty often inflicts hardships on so-called correctly dressed people, their disregard brings exquisite pleasures to the nonconformist.

Since the Bible does not dwell on those bleak days that followed the Fall, it was left to us to imagine how Adam received his order of eviction. Numbed by the incomprehensibility of his crime, confused by his newly discovered virility, torn between dos and don'ts that even to his untutored mind must have seemed inconsistent, he lapsed into a morbid concern for his body, a feeling that not even the most neurotic animals shared with him. The Curse had bruised his mind, alienated his body. "Who told you that you are naked?" asked the Lord teasingly. But Adam failed to see how to put modesty into operation; these matters passed his understanding. Fully to envisage his embarrassment we must turn to Saint Augustine who supplied an important carnal detail on this point. In his *De Civitate Dei* he intimates that erection (the blushing of the penis) did not occur before Adam's fall; it was this "shameless novelty" that brought nudity into bad repute. Obviously, this view is incompatible with Adam's supposed sexlessness before the fall. It merely illustrates the theologians' confusion.

With so much ado about Original Sin we are likely to miss its positive side. For all we know, conditions in Paradise may not have been conducive to eternal bliss. Adam was poorly equipped to resist the steady onslaught of celestial harmonies on his senses and to bear the surfeit of languorous beauty. A man who never had a childhood; who had been deprived of a normal upbringing; who never had a chance to acquire those prejudices and idiosyncrasies that go into the making of an individual; who from the day of his birth (if we can call his strange inception birth) was condemned to permanent leisure—how could he *not* have fallen victim to monu-

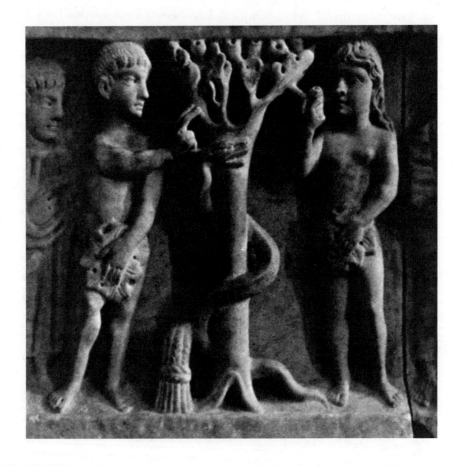

The detail from a fourth-century sarcophagus in the National Museum in Siracusa presents the confusing picture of a still unseduced Adam claiming his part of the apple while holding on to a fig leaf which clearly belongs to a later, post-paradisiacal phase.

mental ennui! Sinning gave him what he needed most: a fresh sense of identity, a chance to quit loafing and to work off his accumulated boredom. We may not be the best judges of his predicament, yet in the light of events it seems that his fall from grace was instrumental in releasing the first stirrings of creativity in him.

Morally tarnished but physically unimpaired, Adam next turns to patching up his and his wife's supposed deficiencies. At the peak of his inner crisis, he sets out to invent a compact little penitential gown—an all-purpose costume so to speak, indeed, the First Costume. (The eternally unfashionable robes of angels, of undetermined cut and material, do not concern us here, as no doubt they did not concern Adam.)

Adam may not have placed much confidence in his first set of clothes, made as we know, from fig leaves. The clumsy, ill-fitting aprons wilted all too soon. But what made Adam turn to the fig tree? Fig leaves are ludicrously inadequate as dress material since they do not lend themselves to being joined together. No matter; apart from representing man's first test of self-reliance and the earliest utilitarian objects fashioned by human hands, it was these openwork garments that made the first couple supremely self-conscious about their bodies. If the garments were identical for him and her —as we may assume in view of Adam's utter unfamiliarity with clothes—they could not have failed to bring out the anatomical differences between the two, and thus opened up exhilarating vistas for playing games of hide-and-seek. It was at this juncture that the Lord, shocked by the turn of events, took matters into his own hands and presented Adam and Eve with fur coats, or what the Bible calls deprecatingly animal hides.

There is a lot to be said for fur coats (and for a more dapper Adam), but what does one make of the chronicler's indifference, not to say callousness, in skipping over a most significant detail: How come he does not mention the animals that had to give up their lives? Or were they flayed alive? Why is the first act of violence passed over in silence?

Whatever the charm or relevance of the various versions of the story of modesty's accidental birth, the fact that they found their way into theological argument and moral precept gives us clues to

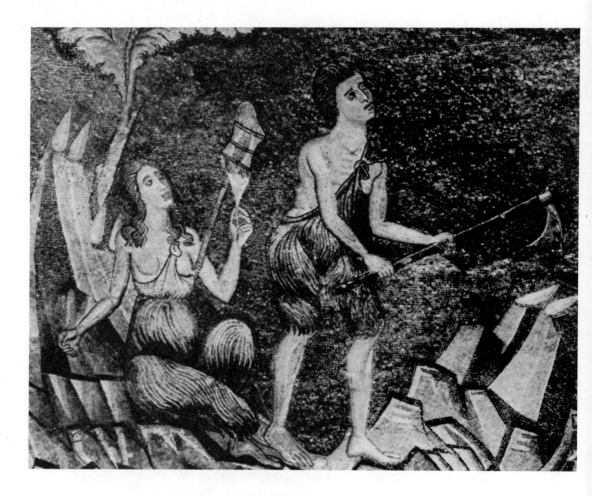

some of our present-day dilemma. The disputes of clergymen, unable to agree on whether modesty was an innate trait of Adam and Eve—indeed the very proof of their innocence—or whether it is a consequence of their *loss* of innocence, have obscured the fact that ancient oriental peoples, including the Hebrews, did not condemn sexual desires and sexual activities as sinful. The concept of Original Sin was invented much later.

If I have been unduly dwelling on the intimate, post-Paradisiac parts of the body, it is because they play a role out of proportion to that of the rest of our anatomy. Whereas in cultures of the highest and lowest level the sight of the unclothed body is considered no more offensive than that of the equally unclothed animal, our middling civilization takes a dim view of it. Complete exposure of the body is thought to be inseparable from exhibitionism, a debased form of sexual gratification punishable by law. Although in the process of growing up as a nation we have come to tolerate the naked body in the arts, in everyday life its sight is still limited, one to a person, to those in possession of a proper license, the marriage certificate. Puritanical society in particular is known for its adherence to Old Testament ideology (which has passed into its blood stream), yet it is comforting to observe that its principles do not go unchallenged. Every generation revises its own interpretations of modesty, and adjusts them to the demands of a way of life that has long been conditioned by Commerce rather than the Ten Commandments.

In order then to have our cake and eat it too, we imbue certain articles of clothing with the power to evoke the same narcissistic pleasures that are felt when parading in the nude. The true exhibitionist acts from a desire to gain sexual pleasure from the emotions —be they admiration, confusion, or disgust—he or she is able to release in a person of the opposite sex. It would seem that this tenet equally applies to everyone who is overly concerned with the clothes he wears.

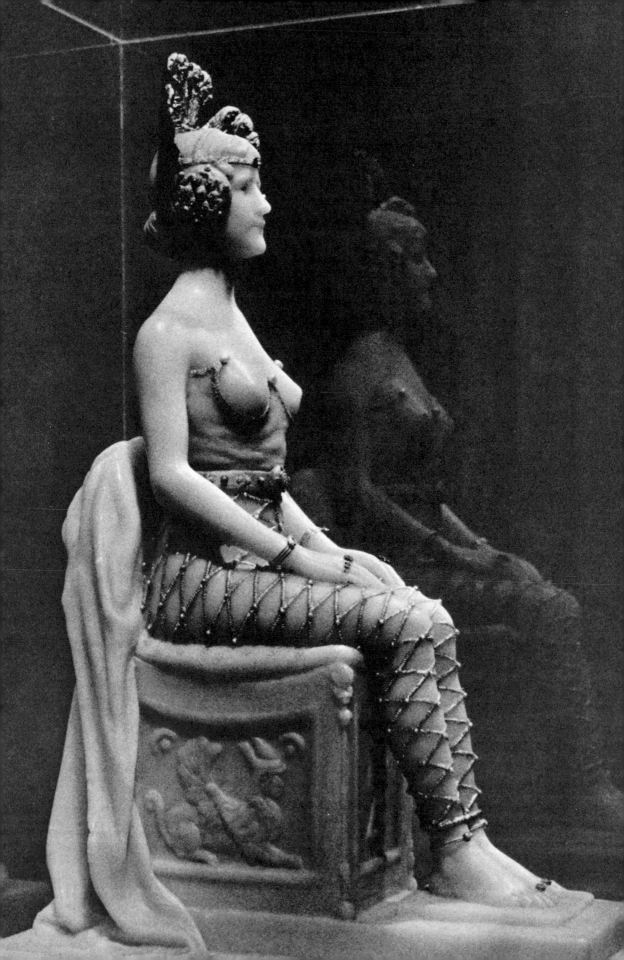

Anatomy of modesty

At first blush, modesty appears to be a virtue as absolute and indivisible as honesty. At least that is what we would like to think. On this point, however, our very language is ambiguous; it does not convey the exact meaning of *modestia* and *pudor,* two distinct qualities which, together, enter into that precious compound that we call modesty. Yet the word as we use it has its limitations. It tells only half of the story; it lacks the rich nuances of the parent words. The Latin modestia stands for composure, unpretentiousness, moderation in desires and passions. Only in a broader sense does it comprise demureness and tact. Pudor on the other hand comes somewhat nearer to our concept of shame. It also includes embarrassment, shyness, bashfulness, and a dash of remorse at its highest pitch. It is shame that we are forever confusing with modesty. "Shame," noted the Jesuit writer de la Vassière, "does not express the real connotations of the Latin term pudor because it is an equivocal word and may designate good or bad shame."

Whichever way we look at it, modesty, or what we take for it, is complex. Put together of any number of ill-fitting parts, it reveals itself in more or less irrational taboos that differ not only with every civilization but often within a civilization itself. Like most taboos,

Ida Rubinstein as "Cleopatra." Wax figure by Stanislas Lami, c. 1910.
(Courtesy, Cordier and Ekstrom, New York)

they defy logic. Moreover, they are highly unstable; a principle rigidly upheld today, tomorrow is abandoned and forgotten. Not that there has been any lack of efforts to bring light into the matter. Anthropologists have patiently searched every corner of the globe for common and rare manifestations of modesty, sifted and examined them but, as was to be expected, failed to come up with any conciliatory view on the subject. Havelock Ellis, who probably has written more about modesty than any other man, saw in it only an agglomeration of fears.

In so-called civilized countries the perpetuation of these fears is guaranteed by the letter (and the arm) of the law. If legislated modesty serves no other purpose, it makes us acutely aware of our physical self, which is of course exactly the opposite of what it was intended to do in the first place. In other words, our brand of garment-conditioned prudery is self-contradictory and eventually self-defeating. To confuse matters still further, a few races show a complete reversal of our concepts of modesty to the point where in some parts of the world only harlots wear clothes. Indeed, the fact that some people habitually go naked does not mean that they

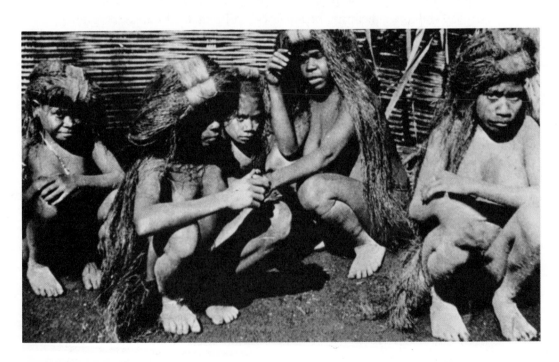

The merits of apparel cannot be measured in yards and pounds; a properly coiffed woman may dispense with dress altogether, as do these wives of an island chief. New Hebrides. (Courtesy, Musée de l'Homme, Paris)

are shameless; as the Encyclopaedia Britannica points out, "among nude races, immorality is far less common than among clothed ones."

It also has been found that whenever tribes accustomed to nudity are made to wear clothes for the first time, they show as much embarrassment as we would feel when asked to strip in public. Hence nakedness, in the right place, at the right time, is not only unobjectionable but *comme il faut*. Moreover, going naked, like going hungry, can be a powerful form of protest. St. Francis of Assisi, an exemplary saint and surely no exhibitionist, once went on what might be called a sartorial hunger strike; "on being rebuked by his bishop, he snatched off his clothes and walked naked through the streets."

Any dispassionate examination of the nature of apparel reveals the unwelcome truth that modesty, rather than being the cause for wearing clothes is its result. "The general connection between modesty and dress," declared Ernest Crawley, "is a subject of little importance, except in so far as it has involved the creation of a false modesty, both individually and socially."[9] In civilizations such as ours which set great store in conformity, precepts of modesty are drummed into children's heads at an early age, yet to judge from the mass of civic and ecclesiastic edicts necessary to enforce these precepts later on, this is no easy task. Once established, however, corporeal modesty seems to be as strong as any natural impulse. It merely confuses by its many-hued facets.

In this country the human body has only recently and partially come to light. Its discovery has taken us by surprise, and many still regard it with suspicion. For historical and emotional reasons in our society the naked body is believed to be incomplete—a body minus clothes. It is the packaged product that we take for the man and the woman.

With modesty's epidermal reaches now distending, now retracting, degrees of clothedness vary throughout the world. Under favorable circumstances—where climate and custom conspire to make life easy and pleasant—questions of sartorial modesty are often reduced to simplicity itself. A single sheathlike garment may confer on either man or woman the distinction of being correctly dressed; no intermediate stages between being clothed and un-clothed exist for them.

With us matters are different. Modesty demands that certain parts of the body be doubly clothed; a single layer is thought to be insufficient. Due to our disingenuous apparatus of dress—a ward-robe ranging from underwear over intermediary layers to outer garments—any attempt to map the border lines of decency is bound to be a hopeless enterprise. To further complicate the issue, conventional modesty is as much determined by a person's station and social function as by the hour of the day and the season of the year. It also varies with a person's age: old men sometimes ignore the most rudimentary demands of etiquette; woman may dispense with the gestures of modesty when their usefulness has become exhausted. Last not least, modesty depends on a given situation. Environment, climate, custom (particularly custom), and ever-shifting laws, all play their part. Sometimes modesty and immodesty seem indistinguishable from each other, and our efforts to un-scramble them fail for lack of a precise point of reference. Never-

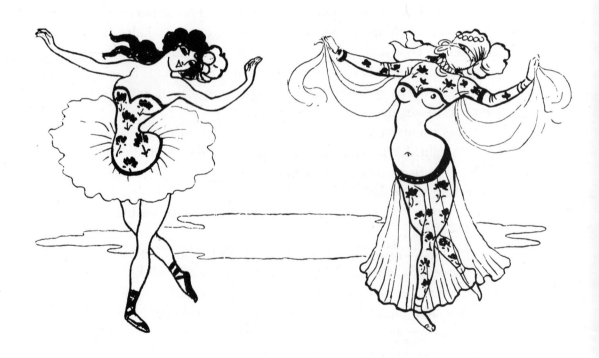

East and West differ in their views on corporeal modesty. Cartoon from Le Rire.

theless, even though it may amount to no more than a parade of national and racial conceits, let us examine the entire spectrum of modesty; let us check the human body limb for limb, organ for organ, for its reputed susceptibility to shame.

It is all a matter of convention. In some Mohammedan countries a woman will cover her face rather than her body when surprised naked. Yet her reaction is quite consistent with the belief that modesty, or immodesty, is written on the face. By hiding it she takes refuge into anonymity. The alleged need to conceal from men what is considered the focus of modesty, occasionally leads to bizarre customs. To cite an extreme case: Family relations in Armenia being what they were in the seventeenth century, a wife did not remove her veil until she had put her husband to bed and extinguished the lights. Since she also got up before him, a man might be married for years without catching a glimpse of his wife's face. (Neither did he hear her voice because, although he was not above talking to her, she was to respond solely by a movement of her head.)[10]

An example taken from antiquity strikes one as no less odd. In ancient Sparta the men were so engrossed in their club life that family life was reduced to bedtime only. The very wedding night was inauspicious for domestic happiness; the bridegroom came home late and left the bride before daybreak. "The practice was continued, and sometimes children were born to them before the pair had ever seen each other's faces by day." Whatever the origin of this cozy arrangement, it doubtless suited a man with an ugly wife. Besides, there is nothing peculiar about worshiping a faceless woman. Our museums are stocked with headless statues, and no true art lover would dream of slighting them. Indeed, few could tell with any certainty which of the dozens of famous Venuses kept their heads and which did not. Just as the ruins of great architecture often are aesthetically more pleasing than the original buildings, so a torso leaves more to one's imagination than a complete body.

Another instance of symbolic decapitation for modesty's sake is mentioned by a European traveler who visited Arabia at the turn of the century. He was received at a princely palace in Oman where the ladies of the house wore diaphanous gowns and had their faces covered with "black masks." They looked at him, he noticed, with embarrassment and, having met his glance, lowered their eyes in shame. Not, he explained, because they were lightly dressed but because *his* face was uncovered. He was made to understand that his naked face appeared to them as indecent as a naked person would appear to him. "They begged him to assume a mask and when a waiting woman had bound one around his head, everybody was satisfied."[11]

The women's request strikes us as less whimsical when we learn that in Arabia handsome men used to veil their faces against the evil eye "especially at feasts and fairs when they were particularly exposed to dangerous glances."[12] Parenthetically, the foregoing account reveals the ambiguity that permeates verbal pictures of dress. Our traveler's veracity is not necessarily suspect; the women may very well have disported themselves in transparent dresses and masks, a combination that to a Westerner suggests brothels and black masses. Yet transparent dresses and black masks are still part of a woman's standard outfit in many Arab countries. As a rule, however, the gauzy gowns are worn over several opaque layers of clothes, an arrangement no more alarming than that of a transparent raincoat over a tweed suit. We also must keep in mind that the black mask in question possesses none of the frivolity of our carnival mask. Still customary from Morocco to Egypt, it is more in the nature of a mouth apron. It covers the lower, least personal part of the face.

Modesty's inconsistency is further illustrated by two incidents that occurred at different times in different places. One happened in Damascus where a pistol-packing mob forced its way into a French officers' club, to protest against the presence of unveiled women.[13] The time was 1945, when the sight of a barefaced female in male company was an outrage to native sentiment. The other concerns a riot in the New York of 1830. The occasion was a ball in a local theater where the guests were stoned *because* they wore masks.[14] The existence of such prejudices in favor of or against veiling and masking shows how wobbly is the line that separates modesty from licentiousness. Indeed, masks and veils often served to safeguard a hetaera's anonymity; "when Juda saw Thamara, he

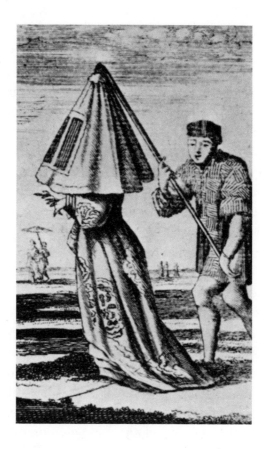

A Nagasaki "woman of quality,"
walking abroad. Engraving from
Arnoldus Montanus'
Ambassades Mémorables.

took her for a whore because her face was veiled" (Genesis, 38:15).
It follows that regardless of what modesty and immodesty stand
for, their attributes are quite interchangeable.

In the Western world the custom of wearing masks was introduced by Venetian courtesans, the patron saints of female fashion.
Here a word is perhaps in order on their little understood function.
Cortigiane are not to be confused with, or compared to, what our
newspapers celebrate as the best-dressed women of the year. With
them the stress was less on clothes than on intellect. They were
highly educated; they spoke several languages, could converse in
Latin and recite poetry by the hour. Some of them were accomplished musicians, mastering many instruments, others were writers
and poets in their own right. Their company was sought by the
great; their liaisons with popes and princes made history. They were
subject to regulations such as wearing a special costume or, as in

Cosimo's Florence, a yellow veil, yet so high was their prestige that their professional badges were appropriated by so-called honest women. (A modern parallel to the adoption of a whorish dress accessory is the vogue of tightly fitting high boots, for ages the hallmark of streetwalkers who cater to clients of ecstatic self-abnegation.)

Venetian sumptuary laws mention masks as early as 1295. By the time of the Renaissance, masking had become a common practice and not only during carnival. Patricians and plebeians, prostitutes, mothers with babes in arms, servant girls going to the market, even beggars wore them in plain daylight. As an article of apparel, they spread to France and, eventually, all over Europe. The French called them cachenez, nosewarmers. Made of velvet or silk, covering the face from forehead to mouth, they were intended less as a defense against inclement weather than as a "raffinement de coquetterie." Some masks came with a handle, or had a button on the inside to be held by the teeth, an attachment probably copied from oriental dance masks. "Ladies hide their whole faces," noted Pepys in his diary in 1664. Queen Elizabeth wore a mask when horseback riding or hunting but nowhere were masks more useful than at the theater where they permitted women to enjoy the ribaldries on stage without betraying their emotions. The last word in mystification was the double mask whereby a person wore a second mask under an outer one, so that when he took off the first,

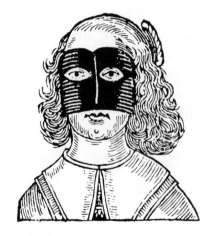 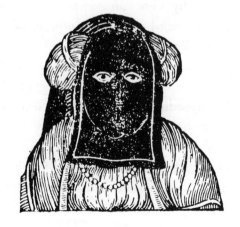

Masked Englishwomen, 1650. From John Bulwer, Anthropometamorphosis.

Turkish woman, 1590.
From Cesare Vecellio,
De gli habiti antichi.

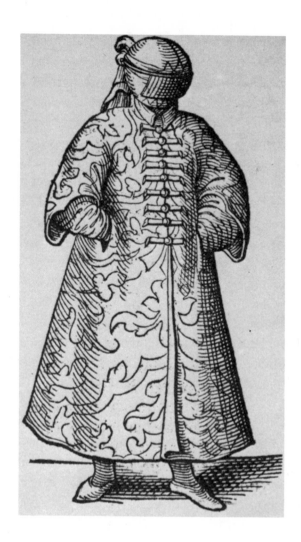

people believed they were seeing his true face.

Traditionally, the priest who hears confession relies on a somewhat similar protection. The tiny wooden screen of the confessional through which pour words that modesty would be loath to utter, is but a stationary edition of the face mask. By unlocking the sinner's floodgates of speech and at the same time sparing the listener an embarrassing sight, it works to mutual advantage. Freud simplified the procedure by arranging the two parties in a way that their eyes do not meet.

Masked or veiled women, it is said, do not blush but there is little evidence to support this view. Blushing is caused by the on-rush of blood into the capillary vessels of the skin, as a result of feelings of guilt or shame, emotions playing on the nervous system. Alas, blushing has lost much of its persuasiveness; the blush as we know it today is only a vestige of a once spectacular phenomenon, the reddening of the entire body. Today an aptitude for blushing, if any, is confined to face, ears, and the neck, and seldom extends below the collar bone. People who blush profusely are so rare as to be enshrined in the annals of medicine. Darwin once had his attention called to a little girl who "shocked by what she imagined to be an act of indelicacy, blushed all over her abdomen and the upper part of her legs." The French painter Gustave Moreau reported a similar incident. An artist's model, taking off her clothes for the first time, reddened over chest, shoulders, arms, "and the whole body." Surely, a non-blushing woman not only deprives herself of an exquisite sensation, she forgoes one of the oldest beauty aids. A blush tends to increase a woman's sexual attraction, thereby giving pleasure to others.

Anybody, man or woman, who hankers for experiencing the sensation of self-effacement with the help of a mask, can easily do so in the peripheral parts of rural Japan that have never or only rarely been penetrated by Westerners. For a few cents he can purchase a foolproof article of camouflage, the kind of mask used by surgeons, which in Japan is worn at all seasons by people afraid of catching an evil germ, or simply to hide a runny nose. This permits one to observe without arousing suspicion astonishing aspects of indigenous life that are usually hidden from a foreign intruder's eye.

Yet true masks are denied us. The only ones we are more or less familiar with are the lusterless muzzles of industrial workers, surgeons, and bank robbers, and those less mentionable ones sported at Hallowe'en and at Ku Klux Klan outings. As tools for instant self-realization they seem hopelessly blunt. Although more people than ever want to improve their faces, the results hardly measure up to their expectations. Noses are straightened, teeth recapped, cheeks and double chins gathered up, yet all these makeshift repairs only distract from the radical and ultimate solution of the problem—the

Japanese farm women from Yamagata prefecture.

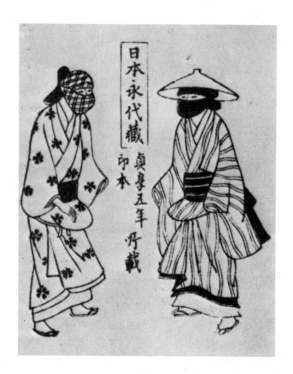

escape into the shelter of a "false face." Such an interim face would seem to be a logical, not to say unavoidable stage on the way toward developing more adequate body coverings. Let us explore some of its possibilities.

It is a fact that nearly everybody, even the least observant person, has a precise, albeit mistaken, idea of what he looks like. As a rule he is dissatisfied with nature's product. He may be unsympathetic to his reflection in the mirror; he may scorn his photographic image; he may reject the portraits he or his admirers commissioned from painters and sculptors because none of them corresponds to the picture he has formed of himself. Although his objections may be unjustified, his insistence on a superrealistic likeness is understandable. He demands more than artistry or resemblance; in fact; resemblance may be the last thing he wants. To shore up his ego, he needs an icon, a holy picture of his inner self. Only a faultlessly constructed mask will meet his need—and his approval.

An unassuming man might be content with a single mask, modeled after his most flattering photograph—perhaps the one he

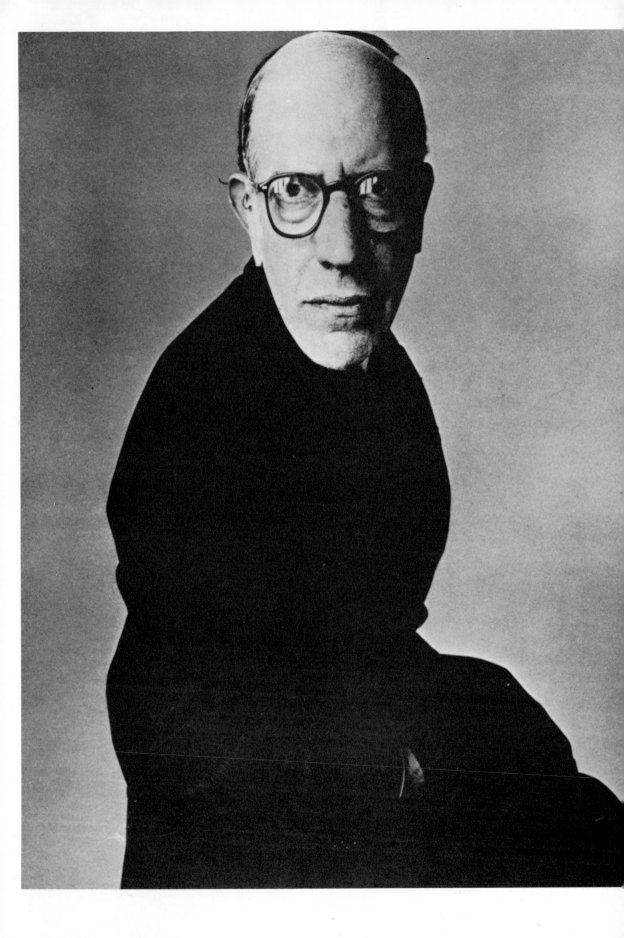

has chosen to accompany his obituary. Or he might settle for an idealized likeness of himself, a sublimation of his ordinary features. A truly fastidious person, on the other hand, might want to own an entire collection of masks, each suitable for a particular occasion, expressing, as the case may be, optimism, indifference, sustained surprise, displeasure, etc., without jeopardizing his basic looks. A person who has been mistaken more than once for a celebrity whom he faintly resembles might unblushingly choose the illustrious face (which would make him seem no more immodest than those immigrants who pick names like Carnegie or Washington for their New World aliases). No doubt, most people would want to look younger; a few, perhaps, older. But rare is the person who is completely reconciled to his appearance, who has never longed to encounter a different face in the mirror.

False hair, false teeth, and glass eyes have been with us since time immemorial, and the false face can't be far off. To mention a few of its advantages: A mask permits anyone to put his best face forward. No baggy eyes, no wrinkles, no five o'clock shadow; all features are permanently composed. At a board meeting, a well-masked man will not hesitate to speak his mind freely, and the steady gaze of his fellow-masks will fill him with pride and confidence. Since few men in the public eye, moreover, are graced with a handsome or intelligent face, a mask can alleviate the discomfort of having to look at them. It has been ascertained that much of the poor impression politicians make results from their visual image. Henceforth popularity votes and personal ratings will be based on a man's compelling effigy. By wearing a mask he no longer needs to show the world his true face. Sculptors, those least useful members of human society, will receive commissions that may decide a nation's fate, and momentous news will be made by the best-masked women whether they wear clothes or not.

The next-best substitute for a mask's protective powers is dark spectacles. There was a time, not long ago, when the country was overrun by what looked like armies of blind beggars. Men and women, old and young, wore dark glasses all their waking hours and in the gloomiest of places. This symbolic, self-inflicted gouging out of the eyes amounted almost to a characteristic of a generation.

Unidentified man, wearing a portrait mask of Saul Steinberg by Irving Penn.
(Courtesy, Vogue. *Copyright © 1966 by The Condé Nast Publications, Inc.)*

Whatever the ulterior motive, whether self-effacement or conspicuousness, whether "good" or "bad" shame (to use de la Vassière's terms), these people, who all had more or less normal vision, tried, perhaps unconsciously, to cushion the visual assault of an increasingly ugly world.

Like masks, impenetrable eyeglasses shift the attention from a woman's face to that part of her body which is, next to the eyes, the most eloquent region of female anatomy, the bosom. The female breasts are objects par excellence for many facetious adventures in modesty. From the generous display of the bosom in antiquity

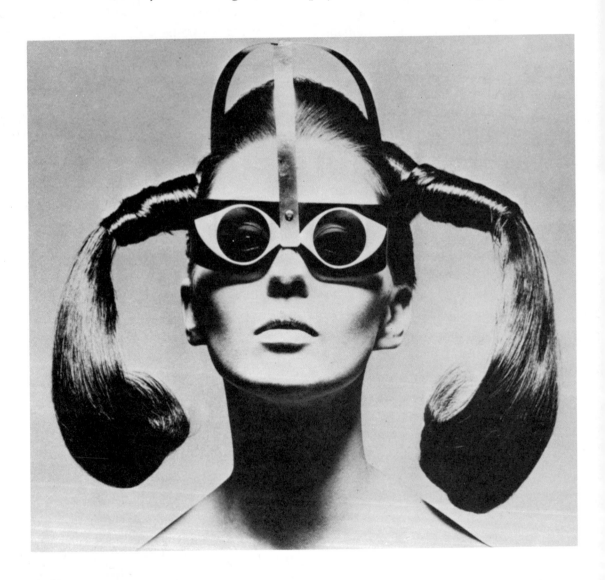

Sunglasses by Mario Marenco.
(Courtesy, Vogue. Copyright © 1967 by The Condé Nast Publications, Inc.)

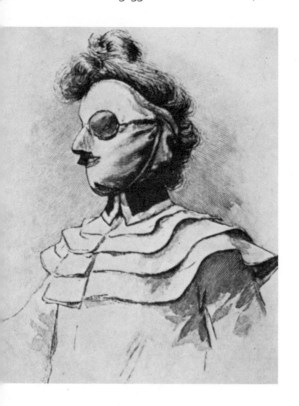
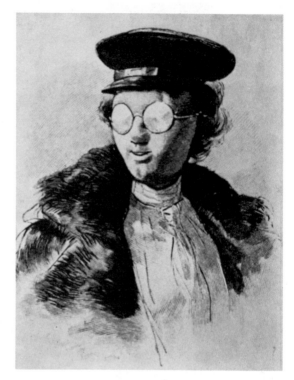

—the *strophium,* the ancient Greek brassière, was intended to steady the bouncy bosom rather than to hide it—to its total eclipse at times when a woman's front could be discerned only by the direction of her walk, female breasts of every description have been much on people's minds. Flat-chested women are favored by some, women with ballooning breasts by others. Yet apart from shape and volume, the love and care of the female bosom, whether clothed, veiled or ungarnished, is universal. Many races, particularly dark ones, still respect it sufficiently to take its sight for granted, although missionaries and underwear manufacturers have done their best to remedy such lack of prejudice.

Occasional glimpses of female breasts have long afflicted Western man with a moral squint. "Too many ladies among us," wrote Dr. Bulwer three hundred years before our time, "who by opening these common shops of temptation, invite the eyes of easy chapmen to cheapen that flesh which seems to lie exposed (as upon an open stall) to be sold."[15] Uneasy as he was about his countrywomen's

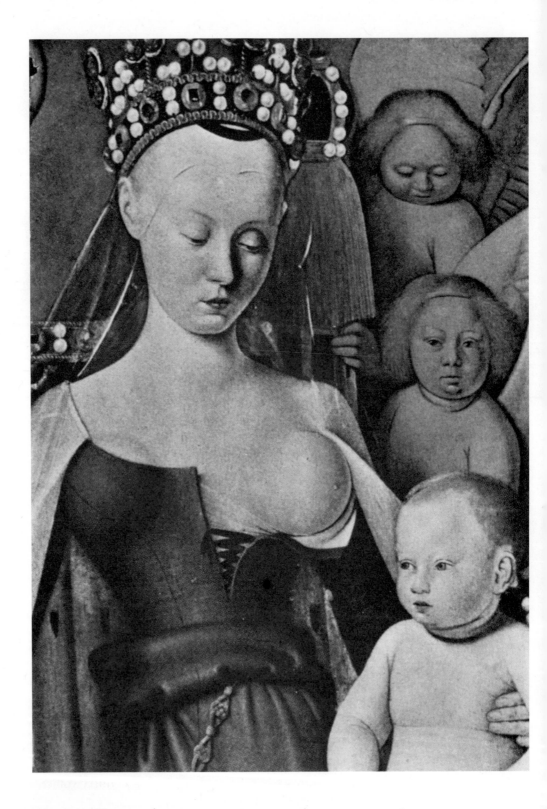

Detail from Jean Fouquet's "Virgin and Child," a portrait of Agnes Sorel, mistress of King Charles VI of France. Royal Museum, Antwerp.

parading their udders (as he called them), he implored them to "shut up shop, and translate their masques from their face to their breast."

France had similar problems. A contemporary of Bulwer's, the learned Abbé Boileau, in his treatise *A just and seasonable Reprehension of naked Breasts and Shoulders*, warned that "the sight of a beautiful bosom is as dangerous as that of a basilisk."[16] (Basilisks, by the sheer ferocity of their appearance, turned people into stone, or as we would say today, gave them a heart attack.) In 1967, Boileau's argument was taken up by the mayor of New York who banned the display of naked breasts in public places. "There is nothing of artistic or cultural value in this sort of thing," he declared in the teeth of art history.[17] The same opinion was expressed more felicitously in a Pacific War cartoon in which an American soldier, ogling a bare-breasted island beauty, sighs: "I'd like to see her in a sweater."

Neverthless, the sight of what the French call the *réservoirs de la maternité* is common in many countries. It is no doubt significant that the fertile, maternal breast is a subject accepted in Christian art. The same Church that at times objected to even the suspicion of a female foot in religious representation—Murillo was reprimanded by the inquisition for having portrayed the Madonna with toes—allowed the Mother of God to be painted with one breast exposed. In Protestant countries on the other hand, to uncover the breasts, whether maternal or virginal, is forbidden by law, except in the pursuit of business or entertainment where nudity or seminudity have long been prerequisites of gainful employment. And although the bosom has been in evidence hereabouts in packaged form, the gallant efforts to break through the brassière barrier have failed so far.

In 1964, when bare-bosom dresses were offered for sale in London —reputedly an offshoot of the topless bathing suit, then being unsuccessfully introduced in the United States—they caused no outcry. On the contrary, women wistfully eyed the novelty; their feelings were affected less by considerations of excess modesty than by regret that the nation was not ready to tolerate bare bosoms in plain daylight. As in the bygone days of dress reform, those who braved public prejudice were ostracized. The volume of sales, however, indicated that the dresses found asylum in the home, the Englishman's castle. There, they clearly satisfied a long-felt need to gratify narcissistic tendencies, or perhaps served to add a bucolic touch to the family circle.

Man, it is said in the *Chanson de Roland,* loves with his heart, woman with the tips of her breasts. Women's emotional urge to occasionally reveal their body is of long standing and was not quelled even in the murkiest of Victorian days. It was emphatically acknowledged many years ago by, among others, the psychologist Céline Renooz. "Women," she wrote in 1897, "have in appearance at least, accepted the role of shame imposed on them by men, but only custom inspires the modesty for which they are praised; it really is an outrage to their sex." According ot Mme. Renooz, it seems that her younger contemporaries rejected false modesty as strongly as does today's rebellious youth. "In the actual life of the young girl," she wrote, "there is a moment when, by a secret atavism, she feels the pride of her sex, the intuition of her moral superiority, and cannot understand why she must hide its cause."[18]

Not that there ever was any lack of females aching to show off their hidden charms in mixed company; history and gossip report many precedents of the British bare-bosom dresses. To recall but one—in the spring of 1749, a Miss Chudleigh appeared at an ambassador's party in what she believed represented the costume of the chaste Iphigenia, ready to be sacrificed. So naked was she that Horace Walpole mistook her for Andromeda. And Lady Mary Wortley Montagu (the sharp observed of the social scene whom we shall meet at leisure in a later chapter) acidly remarked that the High Priest would have had no difficulties inspecting the entrails of the victim. The point is that Miss Chudleigh was no strumpet but one of the Prince of Wales's Maids of Honor, and afterward became Duchess of Kingston.[19]

The latent desire of a native minority to unleash the American bosom cannot simply be explained away as a delayed protest against its long captivity; the reasons go much deeper. A perspicacious lady of my acquaintance traces the infatuation with the female breast to the national habit of drinking milk long after infancy. Non-

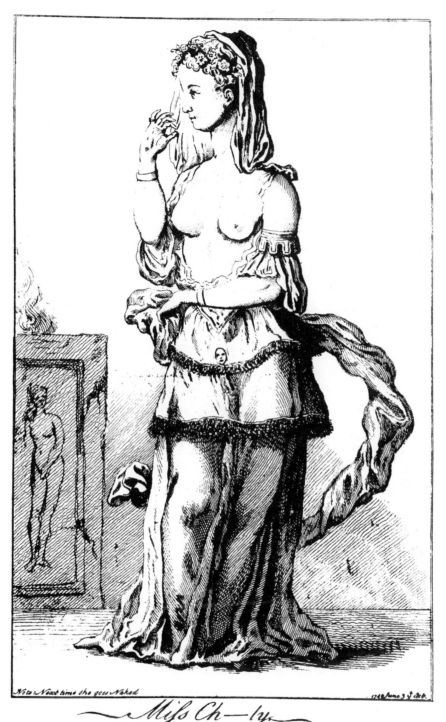

Note: Next time she goes Naked

1749 June 3 J. Cob.

Miss Ch—ly

In the Character of Iphegenia at the Grand Jubilee Ball after the Venetian manner in the Day time; this Dress was Invented by this Lady & the Cellebrated M^rs Ch—r.

Topless female attire simultaneously stands for the glory that was Greece and present-day depravity. Miss Chudleigh, a highly respectable Englishwoman, wore it less in protest against the tyranny of clothes (and men) than as a manifestation of pride. From the Catalogue of Prints and Drawings in the British Museum. (Courtesy, Prints Division, New York Public Library)

Americans find such eccentricity hard to understand. In France, for example, where people of every age drink wine with every meal to promote not only appetite and digestion but cheerfulness and well-being as well; where a soldier of the lowest rank must be provided with his daily ration of *pinard*, the thought of a he-man guzzling milk seems contrary to nature. From a lifelong addiction to milk-drinking, then, there would seem to be but a small step to the helpless adulation of the lactiferous glands.

As far back as 1800, Erasmus Darwin, Charles' grandfather, noted the close connection between breast-feeding and bosomania. In a panegyric on the female bosom he extolled the voluptuous sensations which the babe derives from cuddling up to what he called the mother's milky fountain. These childhood experiences are never forgotten; "in our maturer years," he wrote, "when an object of vision is presented to us which bears any similitude to the form of the female bosom, . . . we feel a general glow of delight which seems to influence all our senses; and if the object be not too large we experience an attraction to embrace it with our lips as we did in our early infancy the bosom of our mothers."[20] Since most contemporary Americans were raised on a diet of synthetic mother's milk, thereby missing the pleasures of playing at the milky fountain, they are afflicted with a lifelong yearning for it.

Banished out of the door, the bosom came back by the window that is the sempiternal décolletage. The last time well-bred Western women bared their nipples was during that elegant, albeit short-lived, period called the Directoire, a time of stylish Graecisms ranging from neo-pagan piety to pseudo-Pompeian household furniture, when women, at least those who could afford to do so, dressed as goddesses and also, for the first time since antiquity, showed their bare feet. The following years eclipsed the female breast by providing a multitude of semi-anatomical diversions. The new century saw the enthusiastic acceptance of a sweeping homogeneous front bulge, a highly artificial protuberance that I shall call the mono-bosom, to distinguish it from the double-breasted chest. It embodied a new concept of corporeal modesty—the merger of two pointed secondary sexual characteristics into a single mass of flesh that has no organic precedent in human history. Apparently, one bulge seemed

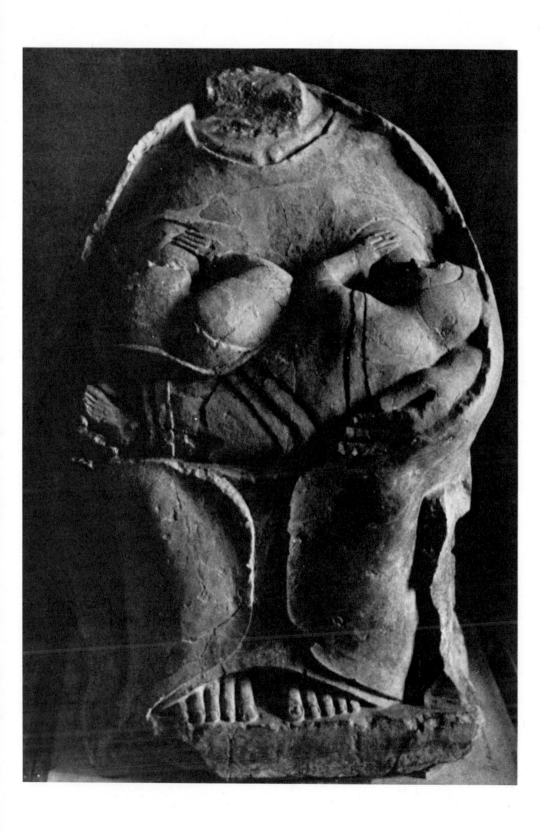

Siculan mother goddess. Sixth century B.C. *Museo Nazionale, Siracusa, Sicily.*

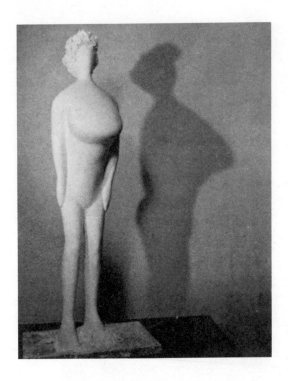

Monobosom.
(See its profile view on p. 123)

less immodest than two. At the same time, a specialized industry made it feasible to mold the actual or illusory substance into variations of every imaginable shape. Quite logically, these manipulations climaxed in the total suppression of the bosom. Shortly after the First World War, its non-existence was decreed, and women acquired a male front. They also borrowed men's haircuts, and assumed a mannish walk. God knows what ever-flowing source of embarrassment her normally developed upper part must have been to a woman.

How, then, did women compensate for the loss of their foremost characteristic? What made them still appear seductive to the eyes of men? How did they manifest their innate immodesty?

The event that, so to speak, insured the continuity of human propagation was the unveiling of the female leg. For five generations legs had led a twilight existence. Only outcasts of society who lived on the periphery of proper conduct, such as circus performers, were recognizable as bipeds. Leg was a tainted word, and in genteel company it still is. Although one does not call a woman's

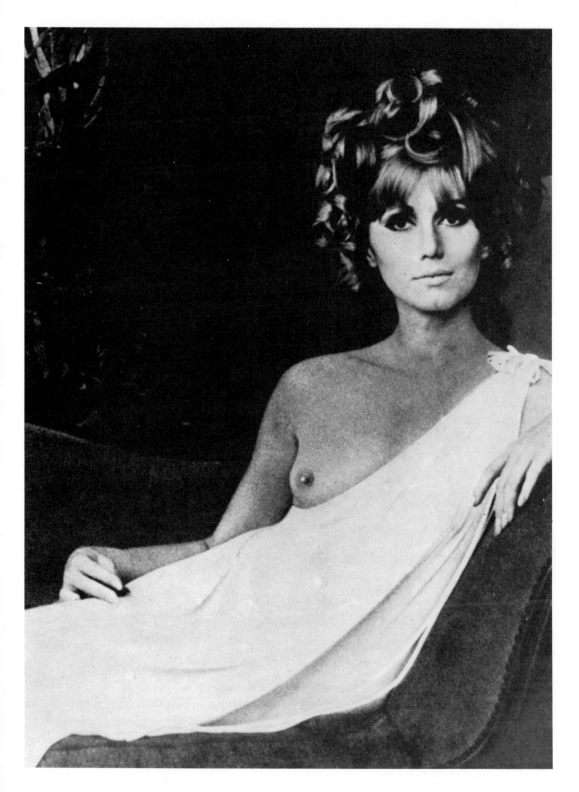

This unilateral décolletage reconciles modesty's requirements with woman's occasional urge to reveal her body. Adopting, as it does, a middle course between daring and denial, its acceptance depends, literally, on the spectator's point of view. Designer: Emma Gibbs-Battie.

leg a limb anymore, a chicken leg is still unmentionable at the table. In this country the philistine resorts to the euphemisms of "dark" and "white" meat whenever carving a fowl; he simply cannot bring himself to pronounce the words breast and leg in the presence of a roasted chicken.

When female legs first came in to the open, it was often thought necessary to encase them in heavy stockings, tights or, better yet, boots. Also actors and dancers, people whose mores are traditionally relaxed, did not believe in bare legs. In Puritan countries, mythological and biblical characters had to conform to the morals of the times. Stage goddesses and nymphs always performed in stocking feet. An English actress "regarded as a calumny the statement that she appeared on the stage barefoot, and brought an action of libel winning substantial damages."[21] Human ingenuity, tempered with hypocrisy, even found ways of measuring modesty in yards and inches. When fashion magazines published charts giving the correct length of little girls' skirts, the yardstick superseded the etiquette book.

PER PATTERNS 2131

the weight of a dress for growing girls ∎nts should be suspended and from the shoulders. ⸬op- Where for any reason her the frock must be ∿ith made in waist and ⸬th, skirt portions, the lat- ⸬ity ter should be made ⸬ar- on an under-waist.

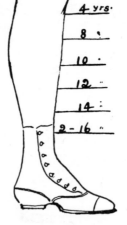

4 yrs.

8 "

10 "

12 "

14 "

2 - 16 "

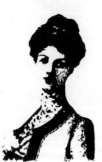

Tʜᴇ proper length for little girls' skirts at various ages.

To our grandmothers modesty was something tangible, indeed measurable. The chart for the proper length of girls' skirts shows the progressive eclipse of the leg, climaxed by its blackout at puberty. Harper's Bazar, 1868.

The domestication of female legs and their belated admission among the visible and mentionable parts of a woman's body was not brought on overnight. It happened in several stages: ankle, calf, knee and thigh gradually added up to the whole. The taboo that covered the foot, however, has not been entirely lifted even in our days. "What's the ugliest part of the body?" asked a 1966 advertisement in an American women's magazine. The answer was feet. The feet of most mature people are indeed unsuitable for public display since years of wearing deforming shoes have reduced them to offensive objects.

At times only the husband was allowed to see his wife's naked feet. This held true for such dissimilar civilizations as nineteenth-century China and seventeenth-century Spain. During the reign of Philip II, women's clothes touched the floor and never showed as much as the suspicion of a shoe. Carriages had specially fitted doors with a collapsible mechanism that could be lowered like a curtain to hide the feet of a dismounting woman. When the queen suggested that female dress be shortened so that it would raise less dust, men sternly opposed such change. They preferred, they said, to see their wives dead rather than share the sight of their feet with other men. Such intimacy represented a strictly connubial privilege and was called *la dernière faveur*.[22] We have the description of an accident in which the queen of Spain fell from a horse and was dragged along by it, her foot having been caught in a stirrup. A great number of dignitaries and troops watched the scene with horror, unable to give aid to the queen without committing the unspeakable crime of touching her foot. When two gentlemen lost their self-control and saved her from certain death, they had sense enough to flee to a convent and there to await the royal pardon.[23]

A similar story, reported at about the same time, reads like a scenario for a romantic ballet, complete with the appropriate tragic ending. A nobleman enamored of his guest, the queen, burned down his castle in order to have the opportunity of acting her savior. Everything went according to plan except that a page who witnessed the rescue noticed that he touched the august feet. The king, upon learning this, personally dispatched the offender with a pistol shot.[24]

Chivalry has long gone out of fashion, yet foot and shoe have lost none of their symbolic urgency. We still throw shoes after newlyweds, or tie shoes to their car. We still hang stockings in the window (or fireplace) without suspecting the custom's libidinous implications. And although fairy tales and folk legends have been toned down to the point of innocuousness, psychoanalysis has given them a new lease on life. Whatever the benefits derived from professional soul searching, not enough ingenuity is expended on its interpretations; "certainly," says an American dictionary, "the broad statement that during all ages and in the folklore of all races, shoes have been a symbol of the feminine genitals needs modification."[25]

Symbols are marvelously deceptive; their equivocal nature is never better illustrated than by the various and often contradictory meanings attributed to foot and shoe. For thousands of years lowly people such as slaves, prisoners, and penitents went through life without shoes, which brought upon them the contempt of all shod people (who equaled wearing shoes with being in God's graces.) Bare feet also stood for a man's incapacity for marriage; "only he who has shoes is a man."[26] Hence our identification of bare feet with monastic celibacy.

Very different laws of modesty apply to female feet. In countries that have not been entirely industrialized, the Church requires women to shoe their feet in places of worship. The precept goes back to the time of the Fathers of the Church when Clement of Alexandria condemned the "mischievous device of sandals" and implored women to wear shoes. We are not told how he got away with this unpopular request when every holy picture made mockery of his words.

Covered feet symbolized chastity, even in Pagan territory. In ancient Rome, prostitutes were denied the use of shoes although no objections were made to their wearing sandals; "their feet's brilliant whiteness acted afar as a pimp to attract looks and desires." By the same token, the Church declares sandals to be all right for monks but not for nuns. Virgin goddesses were sometimes portrayed with shoes, even when otherwise stark naked. Clearly, woman's sandal stands for sexual freedom; it is unknown in Western rural societies. There, the classical gift of the bridegroom has been and occasionally still is a pair of shoes. When the bride accepts them and puts them on, symbolical union takes place. Again, the untying of the bride's shoes—a custom similar to the untying of her girdle or the breaking of the bridal garland—is the ritualistic gesture of defloration. To believe the psychologist, "to uncover the feet of a person of the opposite sex is a sexual act, and has thus become the symbol of sexual possession." Indeed, the word feet is often used as a euphemism for the genitals. Much of this lore has been forgotten, though not enough to completely obliterate some dim atavistic memories. To wit, I have seen a good many Western men balking at the admonition to take off their shoes on entering a mosque, a Buddhist temple or a Japanese house. Unable to account for their mental resistance, they probably felt a sense of emasculation in their stocking feet.

Ecclesiastical authorities are doing their best to uphold concepts of sartorial modesty by telling their congregation how *not* to dress. To preclude temptation in the very place of worship, sermons and printed notices call attention to the perils of exposed skin, male and female. While in plain daylight a décolletage is often unflattering, in the dusky house of God it turns into a beacon that lures men on the path of sin. Some of the warnings are quite specific. One plea, "For Christian Modesty," exhorts females "from twelve years up" to wear stockings in church. Granted that Italian girls ripen early, the charm of their legs would seem to be increased rather than diminished by a pair of sheer stockings. If priests would read fashion magazines, they might have second thoughts on stockinged legs. Besides, how can they reconcile their edicts with *early* Christian concepts of modesty? Have they forgotten that legions of female saints—not to mention the Mother of God—went straight to heaven without either stockings or shoes?

Then again, placards nailed to the portals of Italian churches proclaim (in English) that "gentlemen without a coat or wearing knickers cannot enter." To judge by the clergy's interpretations, the Lord's preference for certain garments and dislike of others is no less capricious than that of any Prince of Wales. Jehovah is partial to men's hats while, according to St. Paul's direction, the Christian God has to be worshiped bareheaded. (Why taking off one's hat expresses reverence has never been satisfactorily explained. It generally is thought to be a survival of a felt taboo, just as removing one's shoes before entering a holy place has been traced to a leather taboo.) Other problems arise from the perpetual changes in dress fashions. To enforce norms of modesty on its own territory the Church sometimes takes extreme steps. For example, at those two great bastions of Christendom, St. Peter's in Rome, and Mariae Nascenti in Milan—the latter simply known as The Dome—admittance is refused to people with bare arms, legs, and thighs. While the attitude of the cleric is understandable, that of the watchdog, the sacristan, is not. Instead of taking a hint from the urbane headwaiter who provides the open-collared customer with a necktie, he drives the scantily dressed faithful out of the temple. Fortunately, the Good Samaritan is not dead. In the torrid summer of 1967 clothing the naked was a thriving business in Milan's Piazza del Duomo. Miniskirted and knickered tourists who found their way into the cathedral barred, gained entrance by supplementing their inadequate attire with rented garments. The postcard peddlers and souvenir photographers who roam the piazza in all kinds of weather had been joined by a flying force of clothes lenders. Ravishing hairdos disappeared under veils and scarves; hairy chests, arms, and calves hid in long-sleeved sweaters, house gowns, and raincoats. The quick-change was hectic since most tourists, geared to speed as they are, took no more than a few moments to inhale the atmosphere of the holy place.

The naked or semi-naked body, so suspect in life, has always been sanctioned in art where its emotional powers are usually reduced to those of a pudding. The erotic numbness that emanates from a perfectly proportioned body assured generations of city fathers that all the mythological statuary that clings to public fountains or dots a town's parks, and the caryatids and atlases carrying sham loads of palace porticoes, are incapable of arousing sensuous pleasure. They would have felt less confident had the sculptors equipped their marble nymphs with wasp-waists and sprouting buttocks. Just to be on the safe side, they did not forget to add the traditional fig leaf. A conciliatory note rings in the apocryphal story which has it that in the vast array of human imagery, the Vatican's collection of antique sculpture, the defamation of the male body was mitigated by putting the fig leaves on hinges. An episode from McMaster's *History of the People of the United States* lacks this suave touch: When Hiram Powers' "Chanting Cherubs" were shown in Boston, the exhibitors felt obliged to drape their loins with linen. "A like treatment," McMaster observed, "was accorded to an orang utang which visited the city about the same time."[27] It has not been reported whether the orang utang blushed at this indignity, blushing being one of the abilities apes have in common with man.

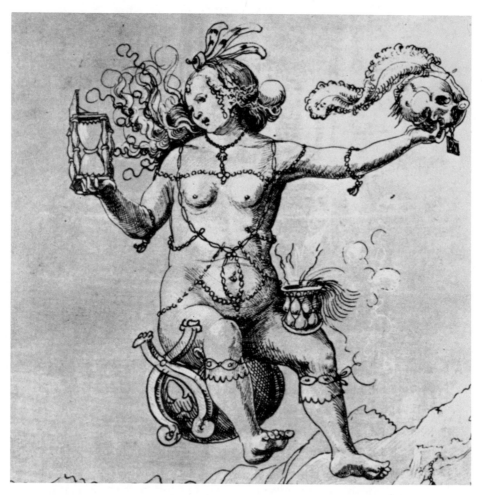

Although stark nakedness may never become socially acceptable in a Puritan country, some baubles and trinkets or a few yards of strategically placed beads may lend a semblance of being well dressed to an otherwise unclothed body. Detail from an Allegory on Man's Mortality *by Niklaus Manuel Deutsch. (Courtesy, Smithsonian Institution)*

The very thought of the sexual parts forever haunts the faint-hearted. In 1967, a baby doll called Petit Frère caused a flurry of protests because it endangered one of the nation's best-kept secrets of human anatomy. The doll, purportedly modeled after a cherub by Verocchio, differs from others by being equipped with the genitalia of a four-month-old male. On its arrival from France, its native place, it passed the test of customs inspectors but ran afoul of the back country's inexorable morality. An outraged Ohio housewife—aided by a committee—dispatched more than a thousand letters to churchmen, government officials, and department store managers, denouncing the "obscene toy." The doll was promptly withdrawn from the display of some fifty department stores but went on to do excellent mail-order business.

Ever since sex was identified with sin, the law-givers who deal with modesty have been concerned with the genitals. Powerless to spirit away the object of their wrath, they tried to legislate it out of existence. Whenever the opportunity arose, man was castrated in effigy. In anatomical drawings the offending member was omitted, and nude marble statues were trimmed to meet the prevailing ideals of wholesomeness. Even wise men were unable to escape the fashionable squeamishness and often gave support to bigotry. Among their more curious pronouncements Freud's stands out: "The genitals can never really be considered beautiful." He was, it seems, indifferent to the fact that his opinion was not shared by many tribes with irreproachable taste, nor that it was never endorsed by any artist worth his salt. (It concurs, however, with the popular opinion that woman is "more beautiful" than man because of the seclusion of her sexual organs.) "The genitals themselves," Freud argued lamely, "have not undergone the development of the rest of the human form in the direction of beauty." The beauty of the human form is of course highly debatable, resting as it does on nothing more substantial than general agreement. The whole sentimental side of our aesthetic sensibility, said Santayana, is due to our sexual organization. Sexually neutral parts are ignored in love lyrics as well as in the arts. On the long lists of female beauty features, from Solomon's Song to modern beauty manuals, the ear, for instance, is conspicuously absent. In shape and texture it certainly

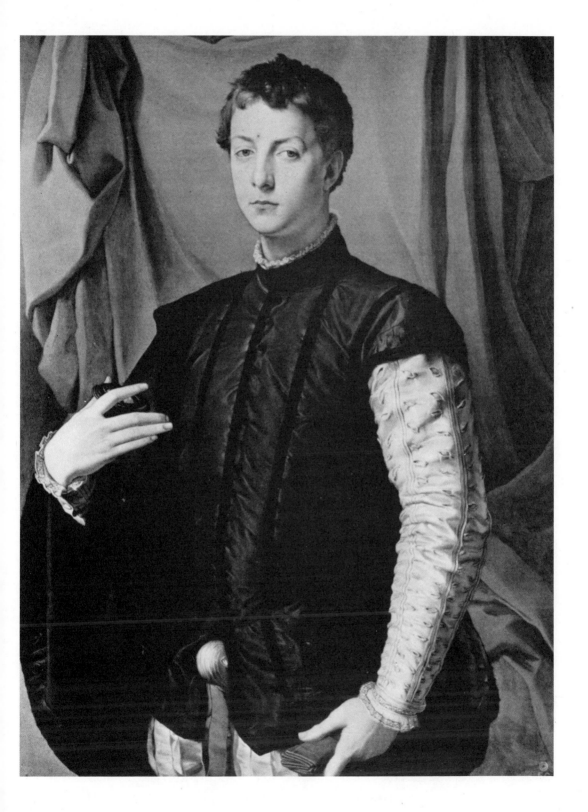

Portrait of Lodovico Capponi by Bronzino. (Copyright, The Frick Collection, New York)

compares unfavorably to the ear of a cocker spaniel or of an Afghan hound.

Although most people assume that the main task of dress is to make us forget the sexual parts, it often does precisely the opposite. Any article of clothing intended to cover an intimate part of the body, sooner or later is apt to turn into an eyecatcher. The classical example of sartorial overcompensation is the codpiece, nearly forgotten in our days of uncertain masculinity. Webster calls it, coyly and incorrectly, a fly. An *American Dictionary of Costume*, rewriting history for the guileless reader, wants him to believe that nothing as evil as a penis ever lurked in the codpiece, that it was as innocuous as a lady's handbag. "The container," we read, "really served to hold money, handkerchief and sometimes bonbons." The very thought of it would have unmanned a sixteenth-century Lothario.

Originally a metal case for protecting man's genitals in war, the codpiece was adopted by the common man in a leather version and ended up as a gaudy piece of apparel made of silk in colors that contrasted with the rest of the costume. Sometimes it was enlarged by padding and stuffing and decorated with ribbons and precious stones. This protuberance was not exactly new in the history of dress; a grossly exaggerated, padded phallus—a remnant from primi-

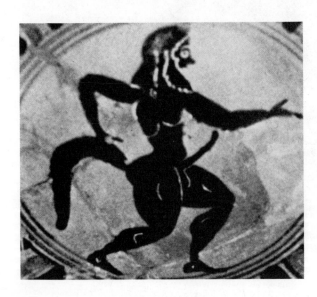

Comic actor.
Detail of an attic vase painting.
Museo Nazionale, Taranto.

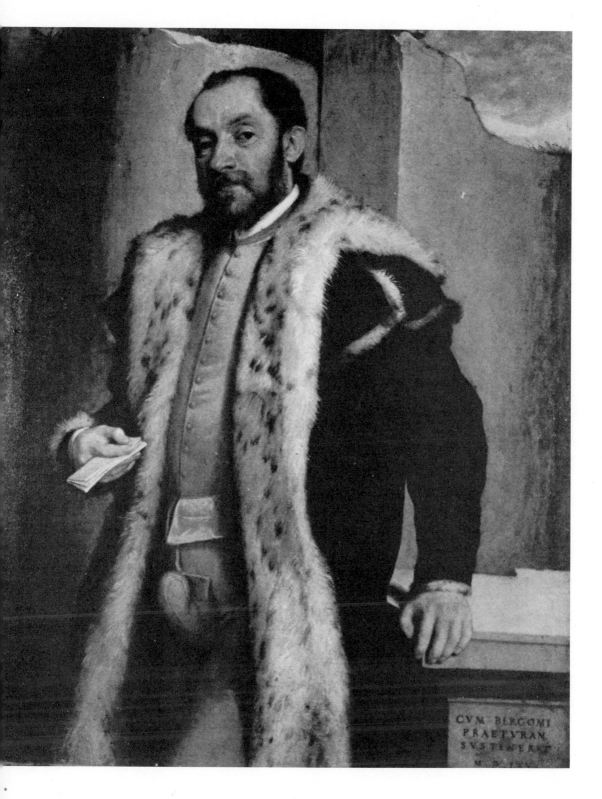

Portrait of Antonio Navagero by Giovanni Battista Moroni. 1565.
(Courtesy, Pinacoteca di Brera, Milan)

tive fertility rites—together with a paunch and fat buttocks once were standard accessories of the actors in Greek comedy.

A homely, if impressive, variant of the codpiece is worn in the New Hebrides where it is the men's only piece of clothing. "The natives," writes the anthropologist Somerville, "wrap the penis around with many yards of calico, and other materials, winding and folding them until a preposterous bundle of eighteen inches, or two feet long, and two inches or more in diameter is formed, which is then supported upwards by means of a belt, in the extremity decorated with flowering grasses, etc. The testicles are left

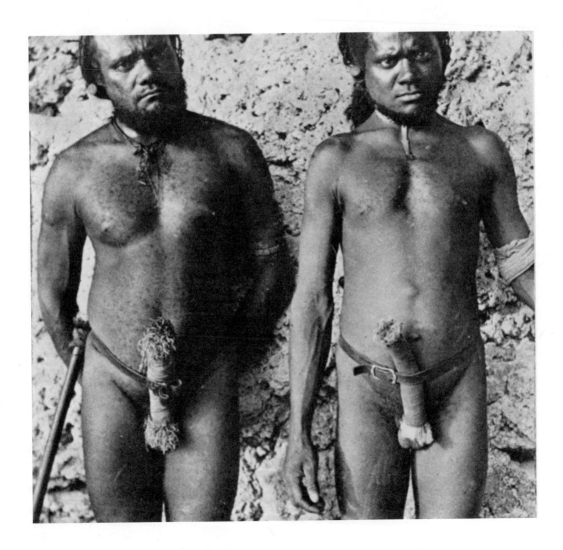

In the New Hebrides, the well-dressed man wraps his penis in cloth to form an impressive bundle, held in place with a leather belt. (Courtesy, Musée de l'Homme, Paris)

naked."[28] A musical version of the codpiece was once in vogue in South Burma; "the Peguans," noted a seventeenth-century physician, "wear golden and silver bells, hanging at their virile members, to the end they make a noise when as they go in the street."[29] Codpieces made of bakelite—without embellishments or Glockenspiel—were introduced in 1965 for bayonet practice in U.S. Army camps.

Today man's genitals are in the doghouse, yet, according to one school of thought, the day is not far off when they will again receive their due. The chief obstacle on the way to their redemption is not the belief that they are unattractive but rather that they seem too unsubstantial to warrant display. However, with our present knowledge this can be easily corrected. Already some years ago, an American women's magazine sounded an optimistic note by announcing that help is now available to the man who cares to improve his scrotum.[30] The method, though bloodless and apparently reliable, may not be to everybody's taste; it consists of the sort of injections used for lifting a droopy bosom. If it should find acceptance, man's private parts may once more emerge, elegantly beribboned and bejeweled, to play their role in the ritual struggle between masculine pride and feminine false modesty. In everyday practice this battle is rarely confined to one zone of operation; display of a single sexual characteristic seems hardly worth the trouble. In order to get results, visual booby traps have to be set in depth.

Modern man's sexual appetites depend almost entirely on visual stimulation; his sense of sight is incomparably better preserved than his senses of smell and taste. Particularly, his olfactory nerves are not what they used to be in pre-industrial times. They have been enfeebled by the all-pervading stenches of an up-to-date environment; the sexual excitement a dog gets out of sniffing is denied to man. (Dogs, with their excruciating sensibility, remain, however, unmoved by titillants such as Arpège and the like.) And yet, the nose, that most prominent adornment of the human face, once was as functional as the snout.

Likewise, industrial man's taste buds have lost much of the discriminating power that is the sine qua non of culinary art, in itself a formidable source of sensuous pleasures. Any man satisfied with

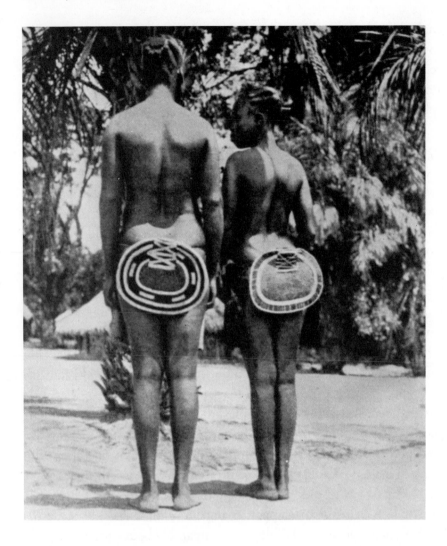

eating the same food year in, year out, finds that a change of diet is
apt to upset his constitution. Luckily for the propagation of the
species, this indifference to culinary refinement is not matched by
a corresponding indifference to human flesh, thanks to woman's
enterprise. Although the exposed parts of a female body at a given
time may be as spurious as the menu at a roadside diner, a woman's
presentation of her offerings is as a rule less erratic than that of a
short-order cook. Having to work with a limited supply of charms,
the conscientious woman never tires to arrange and rearrange them
to best advantage. She herself must have the courage to repudiate

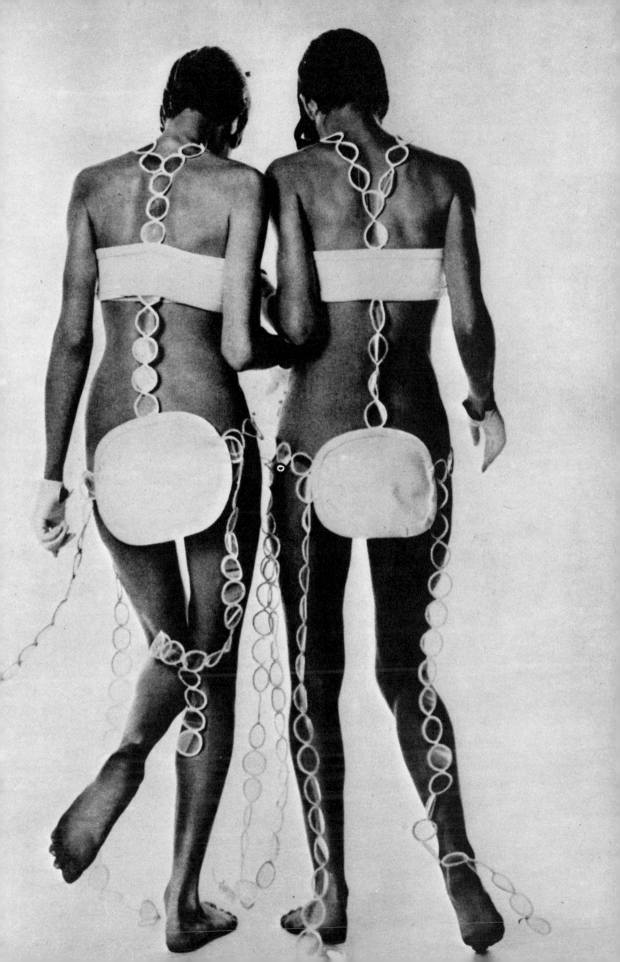

the overfamiliar. Above all, she must never let her attention flag for determining the perfect balance between give and take: On the one hand, since man gets quickly bored with feasting his eyes on a particular portion of her anatomy, she must try to appease his hunger by lavishing ever bigger helpings on him in a sort of continuous emotional assault. On the other hand, to prevent his reaching satiety, she must snatch the object of his erstwhile longing out of sight and replace it with yet another attraction. In short, the active principle of body exposure is variety.

For example, when the (shod) foot came out of hiding, its display may have shaken the moral foundation of many a strong man. But no sooner had he regained his composure than he began to prospect for neighboring territories. To keep him on the right track, and let him savor his discoveries, the hitherto secret regions from ankle to thigh had to be declassified one by one. For the time being the barrier is—at least in polite society—the pubic hair. Unavoidably though, when thighs lose their appeal as *plat du jour,* the curtain has to come down on legs all the way. To recharge them with eroticism, hemlines must forever rise and fall.

In a category all by itself among the accepted ruses for enlisting sexual interest is the décolletage. The strict term once denoted the neckline, the zone extending about two handbreadths from the base of the neck down, obverse and recto. Today, however, it is freely applied to other cutaneous disclosures.

The décolletage is among the least understood expedients of dress; the way we use it, it exploits the obvious while neglecting the more subtle assets of human anatomy. The neckline, the dressmaker's mainstay, is a good example. It is basically a crude affair. Despite, or because of its continued popularity and universal application, it falls short of its attributed seductiveness. Its vagaries are all too predictable. Supposedly a holdout of modesty, it tries to strike the proper balance between daring and reluctance. Although it constantly threatens to overflow its boundaries, it has not done so for centuries; to the Puritan, the odium attached to the nipple is still a formidable obstacle in the path to freedom of dress. Western woman would rather take off her clothes altogether than lower her neckline by the crucial two inches. Whorehouses apart, the Cretan

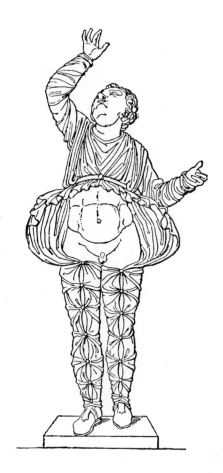

The statue of Attis, a Phrygian deity, illustrates an example of genuine décolletage.

décolletage has remained as remote as the Cretan labyrinth. In recent years, the neckline has come to reach—at least on the beach—all the way down to the crotch (bypassing the breasts), yet such easy gains are canceled out by men's rapidly fading interest. In order to sustain interest, skin exposure depends on escalation which in turn leads to increased bareness, the very bane of the décolletage. Besides, the spell of its accepted forms works only in Western civilization.

A décolletage quite different from the neckline is the cutout. It is based on the principle of a picture frame, or a peephole, and, at least theoretically, imagination is on its side. Essentially a focusing device, it serves, as it were, as a magnifying glass. The smaller the aperture, the sharper the image. Although its function is well understood, it is rarely put to good use. In this respect, the fine arts are far

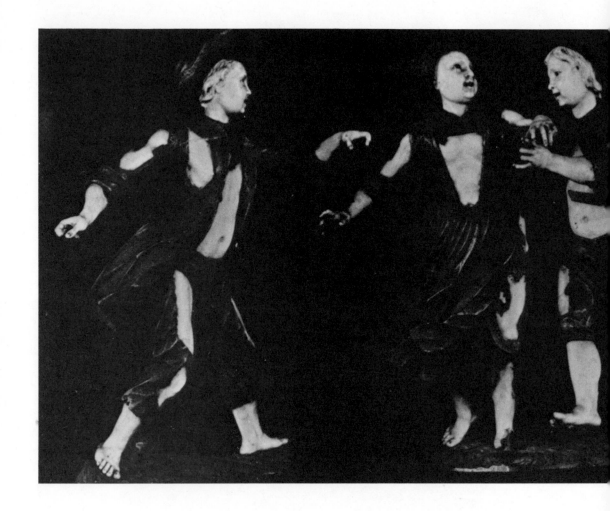

ahead of the apparel arts; artists have applied impromptu décolletage in places overlooked by dress designers. Genre painters with a flair for recording picturesque squalor have lovingly dwelt on the torn garments of street singers and flower vendors, revealing a well-formed female deltoid here, a fragile clavicle there. So far, the garment trade has avoided the aesthetics of rags; in general, dress design is as slick as car design. The selective décolletage, seeking entrance to ever new territories—the rent, cleft, split, chink, and other disarrangements—has yet to be systematically explored. For instance, the multiple windows for breasts, elbow tips, and knee caps, some of which are indicated in the Wild Woman's outfit (p. 66) lie, sartorially speaking, still in the future.

Another means for attracting attention that challenges a woman's

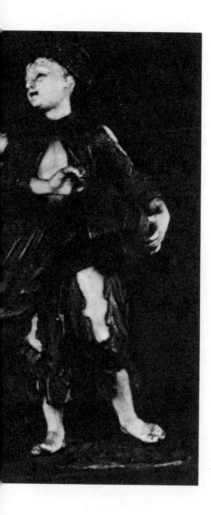

The dancers' artfully torn clothes abound with décolletages unknown in our day. Eighteenth-century South German statuettes of beech wood and ivory. (Courtesy, Reallexikon zur Deutschen Kunstgeschichte, *Munich)*

interpretation of modesty, is transparent dress. I don't mean the plastic raincoat, or the filmy gown of Arab women mentioned earlier, but the veil that clings to the naked skin. It was worn outdoors in ancient Egypt and Greece and, as an intimate garment, enjoyed some popularity in the Middle Ages. It is among the very few body coverings that satisfy the aesthetic requirements of the most demanding critic. In its plain version—uncompromised by strategically placed opaque patches—it holds perhaps the answer to the quest for the perfect dress. As such it was acknowledged by the Greek sculptors who never tired to translate it into stone. Any abuse, however, is apt to injure the wearer. The woman who bares her charms unstintingly may incur nothing worse than envy. Whereas the one who tries to get the best of both, modesty and immodesty, by combining

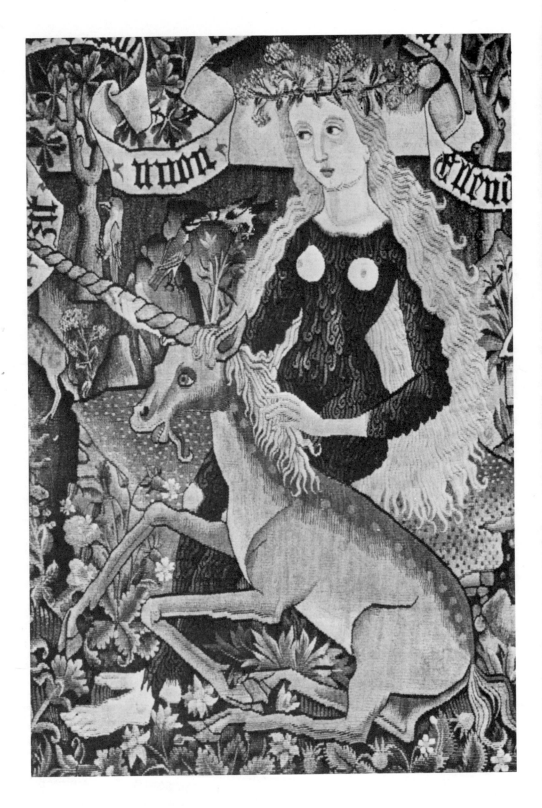

The severity of the Wild Woman's long-sleeved dress is mitigated by cutouts.
As décolletages go, hers are more than a match for our wavering necklines.
(Courtesy, Kunstmuseum, Basel)

Bare-breasted madonnas never offended
the faithful. The fifteenth-century
painter Cristoforo Scacco represented
the Virgin in the dress of his time.
Without the garment's ingenious windows,
suckling would not be possible except
by undressing. (Courtesy, Allen Memorial
Museum, Oberlin, Ohio)

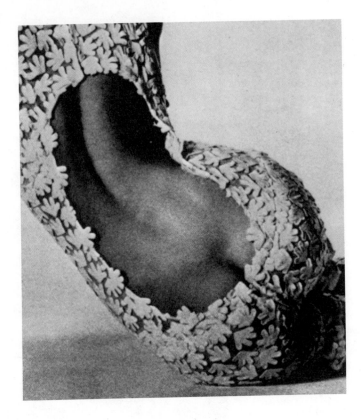

transparent dress with underwear, commits an unforgivable sin. The sight of a brassière under a sheer blouse is an insult to the eye. For the morally insecure and the bodily underprivileged there are after all non-transparent garments galore.

Scarcely less arresting though even more ambiguous than all the allegorical and historical fig leaves is that genuinely modern invention, the bathing suit. The earliest attempts at popularizing sports such as swimming and mountain climbing were not accompanied by the introduction of a specific type of dress. The need for an appropriate costume was not immediately felt, and the first sports outfits were but slightly modified versions of everyday clothes. On the whole, they were beautifully unfunctional: crinolines for the seashore, tailcoats for hunting, trousers and skirts for gymnastics. It probably never occurred to callisthenics teachers that the word gymnastics means unclothed exercising.

With the ebbing of several body taboos after the First World War, outdoor clothes began to look less ceremonious. For the first time since antiquity, bare arms and shoulders, legs and thighs appeared in bright daylight, making exercising less sweaty. When sports degenerated into spectator sports on the one hand, and purely social gatherings such as sea bathing on the other, the human body itself became the prize exhibit, and its display eclipsed all other interests. Sports clothes assumed the role of playclothes in the true sense of the word—an indispensable accessory for that most competitive of games, flirting. Quite logically, denudation stopped short of nudity itself, for an unclothed body is less of a snare than a scantily dressed one. The custom of wearing a bathing suit, a desperate attempt to recapture some of our lost innocence, represents a graphic expression of white man's hypocrisy. For, obviously, the bathing suit is irrelevant to any activity in and under water. It neither keeps us dry or warm, nor is it an aid to swimming. If the purpose of bathing is to get wet, the bathing suit does not make us wetter. At best, it is a social dress, like the dinner jacket.

In spite of its relative novelty, the bathing suit has a history. At the turn of the century, when sea bathing had been declared harmless to health, bathing suits were gay and opulent. Perhaps because men felt foolish about cavorting on the beach, they appropriated the striped tricots of animal trainers and jugglers for their outfit. Women were choosier. Segregated from the men, they nevertheless dressed with abandon, forever mindful of man's secret weapon, the spyglass. On the seaboard voyeurism was promoted from a do-it-yourself hobby to a public institution. Policemen, who have a natural tendency to panic at the sight of an insufficiently clad woman, were instructed to arrest bathers whose clothes did not comply with the official measurements of modesty. Swimming clubs decreed that male bathing suits must reach "not less than three inches from the bifurcation down," and those of women not more than three inches above the knee. Similar rules applied to the length of sleeves. "The modesty of women," noted a contemporary newspaper, "is thus seen to be greater than that of men by about two inches."

Female false modesty remained unimpaired thanks to the invention of so-called bathing machines, the Victorian version of a harem minus its charms and intimacy. "We look back at the bathing machines with astonishment mingled with disgust," wrote the psychologist John Carl Flügel in 1930; "the latter because at this distance, we are able to perceive the erotic obsessiveness of the modesty in question. Future generations may one day contemplate with similar emotions the fact that we wear bathing dresses at all. Our principle clearly demands that we should be able to tolerate nakedness where it is obviously called for, as on the bathing beach."[31]

Flügel seems to have been unaware that bathers without bathing suits had their day within his own lifetime. In the nineteen-twenties, in some parts of Europe people used to bathe in public without feeling the need for a special dress. At the height of summer the beaches on the Black Sea swarmed with bathers who had never seen a bathing suit except in newspapers and picture magazines; their holiday was one of untroubled simplicity. To the best of my recollections, there were no flabby people around; those who ran the risk of cutting a poor figure simply did not undress. The idyll came to an end a few years later when tourism reared its ugly head, and the protests of foreign visitors led to making bathing suits compulsory.

The nature of Dress to Come seems all but predictable. While reasonably accurate forecasts can be made about the development of, say, building techniques or mass transportation, none are ever volunteered on the subject of clothes. Cautious men limit themselves to expressing curiosity about their future, and none perhaps more succinctly than Anatole France. "If I were allowed," he wrote, "to choose from the books that will be published one hundred years after my death [he died in 1924], do you know which one I would want to read? By no means would I select a novel from that future library—I simply would take up a fashion magazine so that I could see how women dress one century after my departure. Because these rags would tell me more about future humanity than all the philosophers, novelists, prophets and scholars."

Would they really? Are clothes truly a key to the understanding of mankind? Do they not, on the contrary, obscure the human substance? And what about unclothed peoples—does their nakedness render them inscrutable? A peek into a fashion magazine (or whatever its future equivalent) of the year 2072 might fill us with dismay. Imagine any upright man's reaction a hundred years ago had he been able to foresee that his female offspring would show herself bare-bellied in public. Would he, in response to such foreknowledge, have killed his breed to save the family's honor? He probably would have had no other choice.

To those curious souls who anxiously scan the horizon for the redeeming "dress of the future," and those no less eager ones who anticipate the much prophesied inevitableness of future nudity with mixed feelings, the half-dress of "a female of the middle class drawing water from the Nile" may look like an acceptable compromise since it fulfills all the requirements of latter-day etiquette. The body is covered from neck to ankles. Only the side view remains exposed,

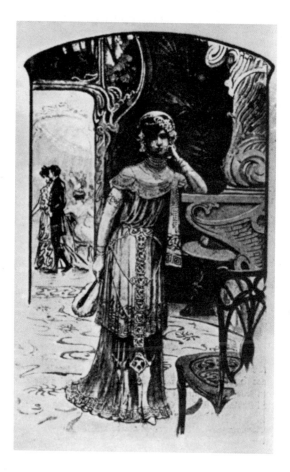
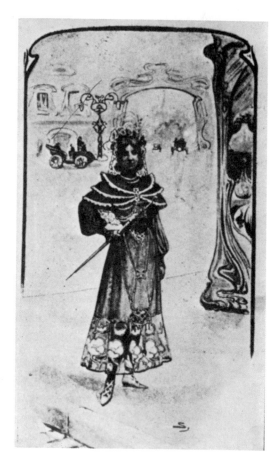

At the turn of the century the liberation of women's legs seemed as far off as that of the female bosom seems today. The two pictures that accompanied an article, "What women will wear in 1915 or 1920," prove the futility of predicting future dress. They also disclose the moral dilemma of the prophet who had to resort to semi-transparent skirts in order not to offend a public to whom the mere thought of female legs was vile. From Contemporaine, *1901.*

but what of it! A mere crack in the shell. In 1851, when Augustus St. John published this picture in an unobjectionable *Oriental Album,* he took pains to assure the reader that it was but an artist's fancy. He denied that he had ever seen a woman dressed in "so strange and fantastic a garment as that which is here represented, open from the shoulder to the ankle, and yet fastened below."[32] Even if St. John knew better, he owed his Victorian audience an apology.

The very same costume is also mentioned in an eighteenth-century travel book by a physician, Sonnini de Manoncourt. The author describes it as "open on each side from the arm pits to the knees, so that the motions of the body easily admit of its being partially seen."[33] Accustomed to the revealing dresses of the Directoire, he conceded Arab women a liberal measure of good sense. "This method of *half-dressing*," he argued, "with air circulating and cooling every part of the body, is very suitable in a country where heavy and tight clothes would make the heat unbearable." (Italics added.)

Alas, we are still far from dressing according to the climate. We are, however, doubtless moving, albeit in a desultory way, toward clothing conditions that, seriously examined, would send unimaginative people into a moral spasm. With female dress becoming ever less protective, physically and otherwise, and with body painting conceivably going to take over some of the functions of body coverings, clothing may eventually turn, if not into the esoteric cloud of legend, at least into a healthy tan. "We must honestly face the conclusion that our principle points ultimately not to clothing but nakedness," wrote Flügel in his *Psychology of Clothes.* To buttress his opinion he cites such fellow optimists (or pessimists, depending upon one's view on institutional nakedness) as H. G. Wells and Gerald Heard, both of whom indulged in a good deal of brooding and wishful thinking about the eventual disappearance of clothes from our world. "Dress," Flügel sums up his own insight into the subject, "is after all destined to be but an episode in the history of humanity, and man (and perhaps before him woman) will one day go about his business secure in the control of his body and of his wider physical environment, disdaining the sartorial crutches on which he perilously supported himself during the earlier tottering

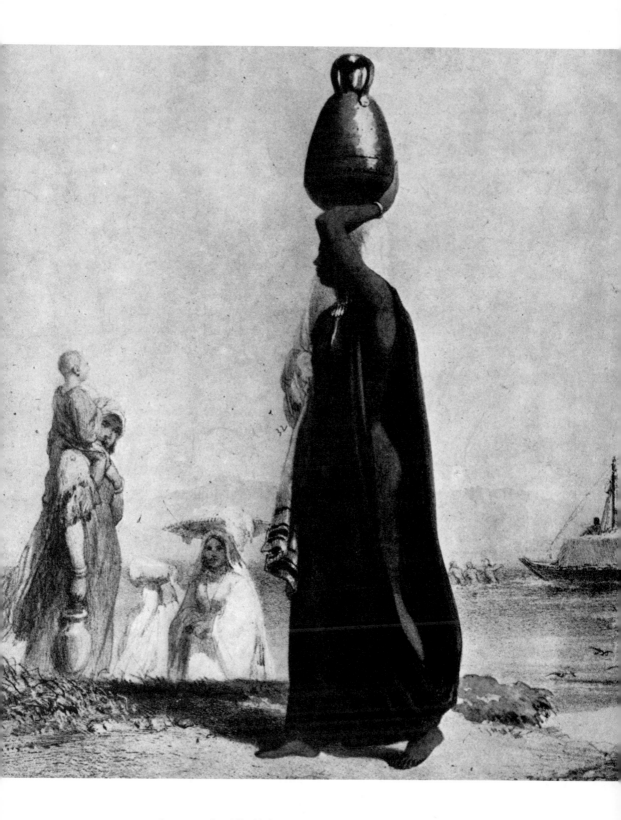

An example of "half-dress" from the Oriental Album *by James Augustus St. John.*

stages of his march towards a higher culture."

Some forty years ago when these words were written such conjectures sounded perhaps less naïve than they do today. Flügel's England and the European continent have hardly progressed toward "a higher culture." In the United States of today nudity is taken for granted on the printed page and on the stage but as yet has not received the (posthumous) blessings of Emily Post, still less those of the law. It is associated with San Francisco rather than Saint Francis. Yet nakedness has always been at home in so-called dark continents. When Flügel spoke of "humanity" he conveniently ignored those Asian and African nations to whom going more or less naked never presented moral qualms. People who traditionally do not have much use for clothes are not amused by the missionary zeal that prompts us to press our notions of decency upon them while being insensitive or opposed to theirs. It would take a moral sandblasting to rid ourselves of the layers of false modesty we accumulated through the centuries.

An instructive example for pointing up the many inconsistencies in regard to modesty can be found in Japan where until about one hundred years ago most customs ran counter to those in the Western world. In fact, even today, after spectacular changes, the Japanese have remained skeptical about our morals, as indeed we have about theirs. While we are willing to admire their ethics and aesthetics as expressed in works of art, we draw the line at their domestic manners. Until recently, their attitude toward the human body was the exact opposite of ours: The nude was seen in daily life but inadmissible in traditional art. Artists showed no interest in rippling muscles and swelling bosoms; they invariably portrayed people dressed to the nines. Even lovers, bedded down on acres of quilts—a favorite subject in art—are always fully clothed, not because the artists were prudes but because the Japanese seem to like making love entangled in each other's garments. "Unforgettably horrible is the naked body," wrote Lady Murasaki, the author of the *Tale of Genji;* "it really has not the slightest charm." Probably for that very reason nakedness at home, at the bathhouse or inn, was, and still is, anything but to be avoided except in the presence of a foreigner with an evangelical turn of mind.

One might add that from an aesthetic point of view, Japanese nudity is far more attractive than ours because their bodies are hairless, and, before affluence caught up with them, they never exhibited the sad effects that betray our superior standard of living—paunches, garlands of fat, and deformed feet. (A blind masseur can tell a Westerner from a Japanese by merely touching his toes.) Best of all, the Japanese are able to preserve a youthful body far into old age. Being descended as they are directly from the gods, they not only skipped Original Sin but also never felt a need for adopting it. Despite a strong desire to make every one of our prejudices their own, they did not succeed in acquiring a fear of nakedness.

In general, that part of mankind that has kept its wits about it, has proved unreceptive to our morals; where the climate is favorable, the belief in the integrity of the naked body remains intact. Hence we still find in foreign countries clothing conditions that, transplanted to our own environment, seem sheer utopia. Unfortunately, our superiority complex does not allow us to share other peoples' wisdom. If we insist on being guided by our heritage of guilt and fear, we shall have to go a long way toward an unbiased view of nakedness. Dunlap Knight, writing on costume, neatly summed up our predicament: "In modern civilization there has grown up an immodesty which was lacking in more ancient cultures. We are ashamed of our bodies. Whether the practice of concealing the body is the cause of our uncleanliness of mind, or whether our obscenity is rather the cause of concealment, is a debated question."[34]

To the caveman-painter the shape of the human figure seems to have been just as boring as it is to today's artist. It mainly served him as a theme for endless variations. Prehistoric cave drawings, Spain. From Abbé Breuil's *Anthropologie*.

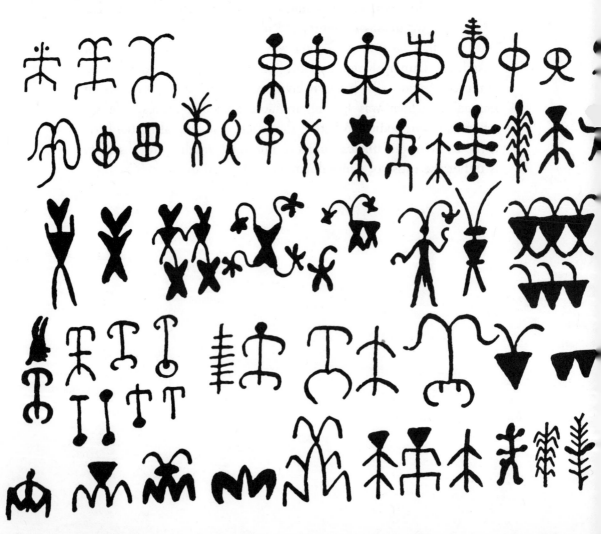

A portfolio of monsters

To say that people come in all shapes and sizes is gross exaggeration; lean or fat, short or tall, they look depressingly alike. Barring a quirk of nature or some misfortune, they all have the same kind of trunk, the same extremities in the same places, and move more or less in the same way. Hence man's boredom with his body, his fascination with giants and dwarfs, with the bearded lady.

Strip mythology and folklore, poetry and art of their monsters and you are left with an impoverished universe. Helias' fauns and nereids; India's many-limbed deities; Bosch's ghoulish melting pot; Shakespeare's "men whose heads do grow beneath their shoulders"[35] —how can the world do without them! One only has to scour the Egyptian Sky or the Greek Olympus for godly and ungodly creatures to realize what prominent part monsters played in man's imagination. Not that his imagination has worked wonders. For all their otherworldliness these monsters are eclectic, assembled from fragments of man and beast. Indeed, so elementary is their structure that anybody with half a sense of the bizarre is able to piece them together by easy-to-follow instructions.

The basic ingredients for Greek monsters are, roughly, choice specimens of man, woman, lion and horse; a bull's head, one or two fish tails, a pair of goat legs, a couple of feathery wings, a basket-full of serpents and, perversely, a tree trunk. These disparate components have been synthetized with impeccable taste into classical clichés: A man with a bull's head becomes a minotaur, a horse with a man's head a centaur, a woman-headed lion makes a she-sphinx (as distinct from the Egyptian Great Sphinx of Giza which is male), a fish-tailed woman is known as a siren, a goat-footed man as a satyr, and so forth, each combination attaining a new identity. The only attempt to escape these zoomorphic permutations is exemplified by Apollo's love, Daphne, whose mother magically transformed her body into

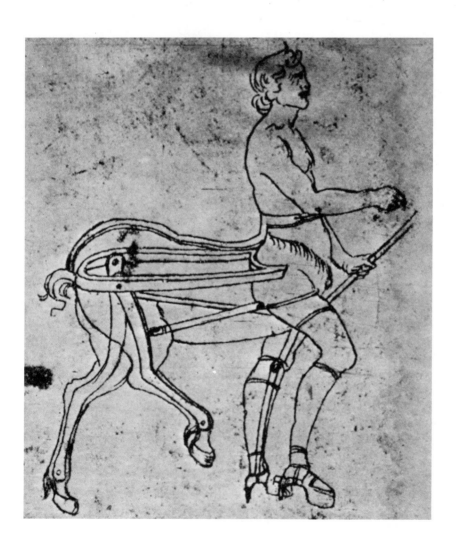

Design for a stage centaur by Francesco di Giorgio.
Collection Fairfax Murray, London.

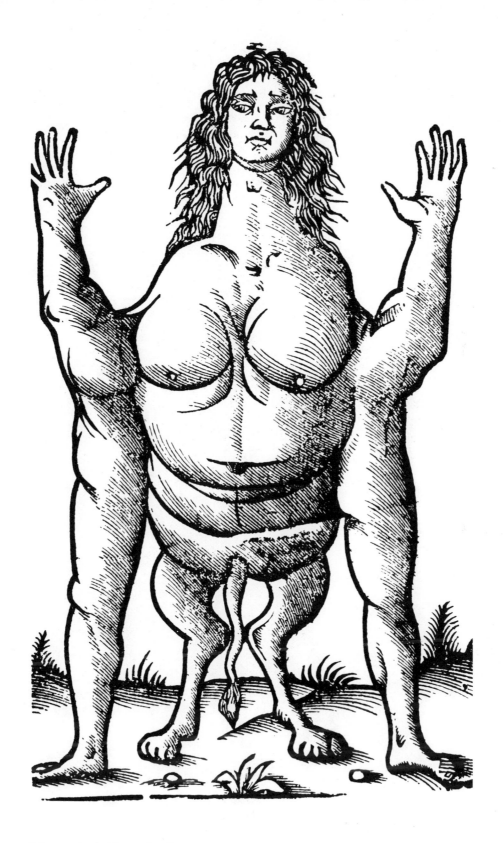

Monster from Alessandro de' Vecchi,
Aggiunta alla quarta parte dell' Indie, etc., 1623

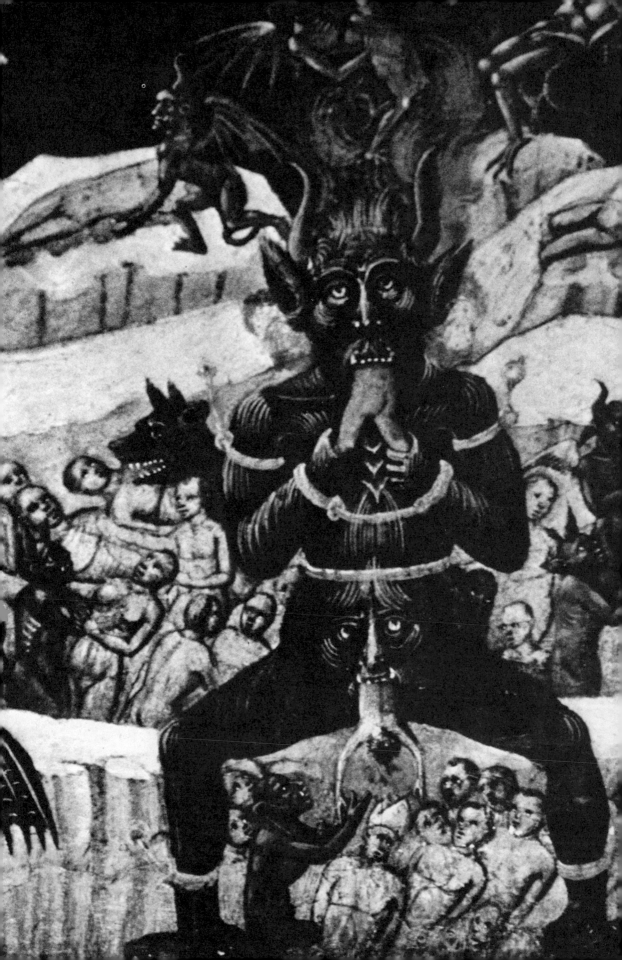

a laurel tree. A similar scrambling of bodies and limbs produced ancient Egypt's glut of sacred monsters. The Nilotic deities—images of men and women with the heads of ape, bull, falcon, hawk, ibis, jackal, lion and ram—never leave their terrestrian bounds. Piety is in a rut, not since prehistoric times has man come up with anything new in the way of idols.

Christianity, a heavy borrower from the doctrines of antiquity, sometimes accepted heathen fixtures on probation. Exercising a calculated tolerance of man's darker fantasies, it did little to depreciate monsters. Quite the contrary; it often provided a niche for them under the portals of churches and convents where stony rows of grossly abnormal creatures share and, it would seem, enhance the company of saints and angels. Others, perching high on cathedral roofs, alternate with chimeras and gargoyles, while altarpieces give asylum to a netherworld of beings that one would hate to encounter in one's dreams.

What beneficial influence flowed from these works of art, apart from shoring up the fear of God and Satan? Did they not rather have an adverse effect on the pious? To be more specific—was it possible that an expectant mother would take fright at the sight of the diabolical images and, as a consequence, give birth to a monster? The Church might deride such conjectures yet, from a sense of duty, and mindful of the mother's salvation, burn her at the stake. What posed a problem was the baby monster. Learned men differed in their opinions whether to consider him human or not, opinions which decided his chances for receiving the spiritual consolations of religion. Mercifully, the majority thought him deserving of their ministrations; in one *Sacred Embryology*, published in 1745, its author, the inquisitor of the kingdom of Sicily, devoted an entire chapter to the baptism of monsters.

Monstrous creatures of every description have a long past. According to the Bible, "there were giants on the earth" (Gen. VI, 4) yet the untidy accounts do not mention at what point and for what purpose they were created. Medieval theologians regarded them as the children of fallen angels, and doubtless there has always been an aura of evil attached to them. They are usually referred to as ill-clothed, man-eating and rock-hurtling, although when in a peaceful

The memory of the ancient monsters has been perpetuated by religious art. Centaurs (see p. 256), flying dragons, and human-headed serpents (p. 257) abound in the figurative arts, from illuminated manuscripts to monumental altar pieces. The man-eating devil in Bologna's San Petronio has cowed twenty generations of worshipers.

mood, they were capable of performing such chores as building cyclopic walls of unsurpassed workmanship. However, it is their dress rather than their manual feats that staggers the imagination. Picture if you will a loincloth whose dimensions run to several hundred feet, the size of a Sassanian carpet, or try to guess the weight of Goliath of Gath's armor! Yet, Goliath represented only a mild case of glandular unbalance. Although his eleven-foot five-inch frame would look impressive in today's low-ceilinged apartments, he was small fry compared to the high-rise giants of his time. The Israelites of the Exodus, one reads, "seemed as grasshoppers by the side of the Anakim."

Apart from giants there also were super-giants. The biblical Og— not to be confused with the London-based giants Gog and Magog— was several miles tall. With his head in the clouds, walking must have been hazardous to him. But then, all colossal beings shared the same problem; a very distant tribe, Mexican giants, used to greet each other with "Fall not, for who falls, falls forever." At any rate, giants came early to grief and vanished like their animal counterpart, the dinosaurs. They probably were too expensive for nature to feed.

Accepting as we do religion's giants on pure faith—only one of them, Christopher the Christ-bearer, was admitted to the court of saints—we cannot very well afford to question the disclosures of science. The enormous jaws, teeth and thighbones that were dug from the soil are every bit as much proof of a fabulous past as Schliemann's gold. Unfortunately, posterity has played fast and loose with them. What, for instance, became of the "perfect skeleton" of a man measuring four hundred feet, found through one of those rare strokes of luck on Mount Erice in western Sicily? It was rescued from oblivion by the renowned seventeenth-century mathematician and archaeologist Athanasius Kircher who included its description in his magnum opus *Mundus Subterraneus*. An accompanying engraving shows the giant towering above the infinitesimal *homo ordinarius*. Surely, the residual bones of a creature the height of a forty-story building should have been worth preserving, all the more so as Kircher surmised them to be those of the famous Cyclop Polyphemus himself.

Giants having shown an early tendency of becoming extinct—

already Homer lamented the disappearance of men of great stature —man's interest turned to the other extreme, dwarfs. The imps, elfins, kobolds, and trolls of mythology have their earthly counterpart in the little people who make up a minuscule part of humanity. Malformed or well-proportioned, it was their fate to be treated as sort of domesticated goblins and, since they take up less space than giants, they became collectors' items. Like pet animals, they were elevated to household ornaments and status symbols by those who could afford them. The Romans, particularly, were fond of pint-size humans. Marc Anthony, Augustus and Tiberius sought the company of dwarfish jesters "to relieve the languid hours." (The last vestige of this sort of entertainer is the ventriloquist's dummy.)

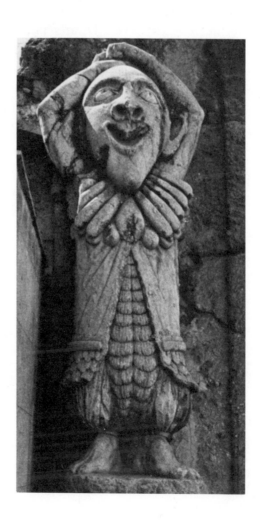

Stone figure of a court jester in the Villa Palagonia, Bagheria, Sicily.

Emperor Diocletian, an aficionado of the circus and the theater, kept a stable of miniature gladiators, fleshed-out puppets of faultless articulation. "These and similar varieties of the human race," commented Pliny the Elder with chilling unconcern, "have been made by the ingenuity of Nature as toys for herself and marvels for us."

Throughout history, the names and faces of these dwarfs were as well known as those of today's comedians, and none better than the buffoons of the Spanish court. Such was their eminence that kings and princes had them portrayed by the great masters of the time. Velásquez immortalized no less than seven dwarfs attached to Philip the Fourth's household. His most celebrated work, "Las Meninas," shows Mari Bórbola and Nicolasito Pertusato, the playthings of the Infanta. (Would anybody blame a child for bestowing his affection on the Seven Dwarfs rather than on his guardian angel?) Philip's successor, Charles II, who upheld the tradition of portraying the melancholy little creatures, was so amused by the deformed Eugenia Martinez Vallejo that he ordered the court painter Carreño de Miranda to paint her in the nude. Today her picture hangs in the Prado.

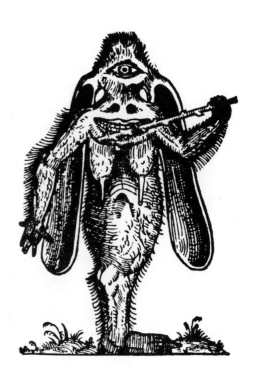

Cyclop, sea monk, *and sea bishop,*
from Recueil de la diversité des habits, *1562.*

Not always, however, did dwarfs have to make a living as pages and jesters. There were scholars and artists, even soldiers among them, yet the popular belief that they were made by the devil died hard. "Even as sometimes dwarfs and giants may be naturally procured," wrote the afore-mentioned Dr. Bulwer, "so the devil with more facility can, by divine permission, promote the decrease or increase of the human stature, by applying Actives and Passives."[36] Strictly speaking, dwarfs and giants are purely quantitative aberrations of nature; they do not intrigue us as much as the physically scrambled monsters. For all his elephantine size and the single eye in the middle of his forehead, Polyphemus was no match for, say, the Four-eyed Man of Cricklade, the *lusus naturae* mentioned by Drury. Not only had this man perfect vision in everyone of his eyes, he could revolve them separately in their orbits, and close any particular one while keeping the others open.

Although the old myths have long been replaced by modern ones, man's fascination with monsters did not abate in the Age of Enlightenment. The sixteen figures on pp. 86 and 87, reprinted from woodcuts in Schedel's 1493 *Liber Chronicarum*, are scarcely less

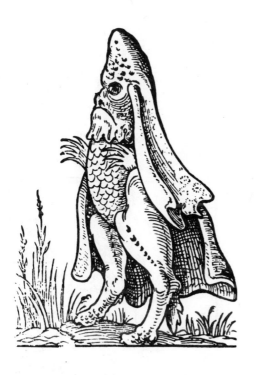

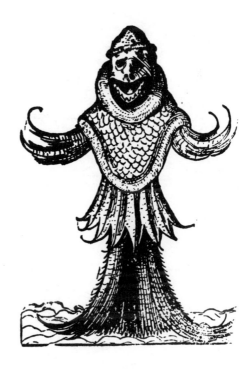

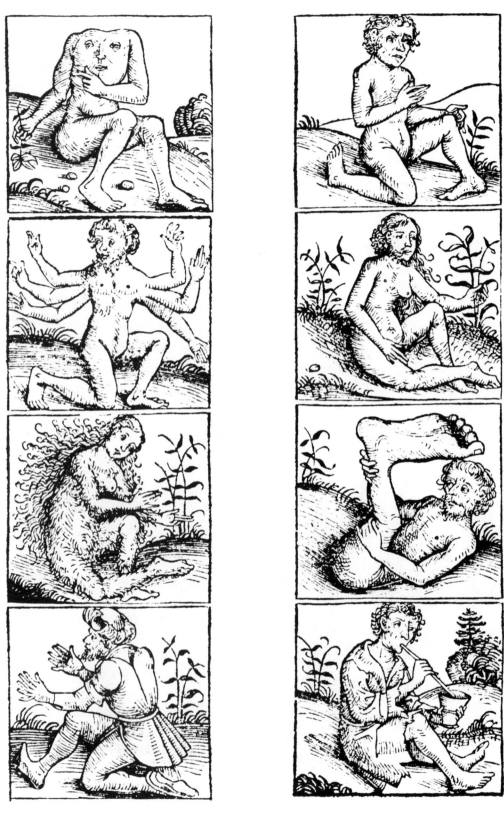

At a time when information was even less reliable than it is today, people with four eyes, six arms, or ears long enough to serve as couch and cover, were believed to be an odd but pleasant reality.

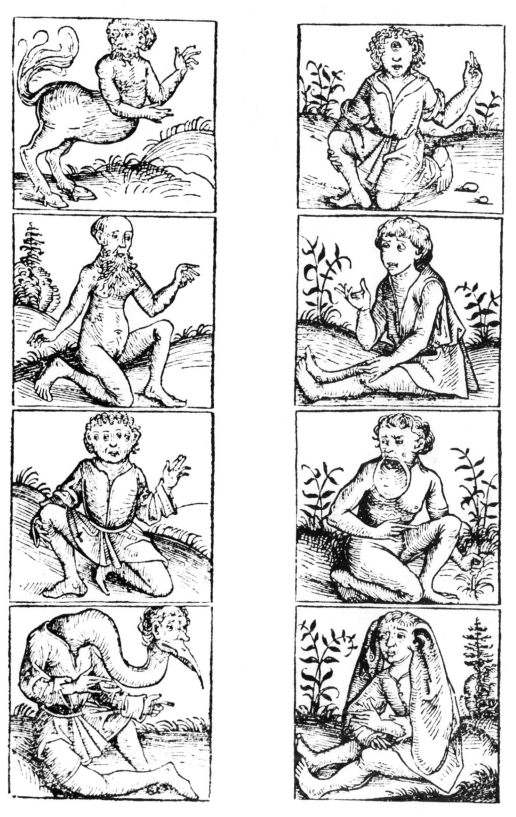

The woodcuts, reproduced from Hartmann Schedel's Liber Chronicarum. *1493, do not represent individual monsters but stand for so many races or nations.*

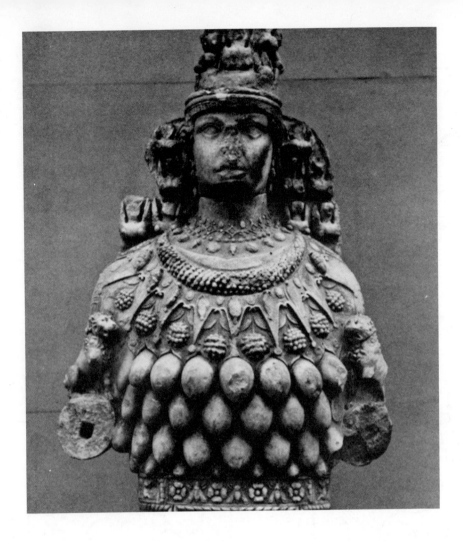

arresting, if admittedly a good deal more ambiguous, than the divine monsters of antiquity. They are based on the seventh book of Pliny's *Natural History* whose subject is Man. What makes them doubly interesting is the fact that they do not just represent—as one might think from a glance—a few unique individuals but are meant to typify some of mankind's races. Who ever believed, Pliny wrote, in the Ethiopians before actually seeing them! Although he was a traveler in his own right, he does not imply that he ever encountered the strange men and women he describes with so much relish. He drew instead on an inexhaustible supply of information and quoted at length, though not always with conviction, a host of Roman and foreign authors.

Upon closer inspection, these monsters turn out every bit as

posite: While supernumerary nipples are not uncommon in both male and female
sons, rows of them belong to mythology. The many breasts of the Ephesian
temis symbolize her role as the all-nourishing mother.

baffling as the ancient ones, if not more so. Among the "nations" which Pliny describes we meet Indian pygmies who build houses from eggshells, feathers, and mud. Others, such as the one-legged Monocoli, move by jumping with great speed; "They are called the Umbrella-foot tribe because in the hotter weather they lie on their backs on the ground and protect themselves with the shadow of their feet."[37] Still another Indian region is inhabited by people who, although their feet are turned backward, run extremely fast. Dearth of evidence is often compensated by a touch of poetry. Thus we are told that the Astomi who live near the sources of the Ganges have no mouth; they subsist on air and the fragrance of fruit and flowers. On long journeys they carry wild apples with them so as not to run out of a supply of scent, and so sensitive are they that strong, unusual odors will kill them. The *Liber's* collection of aberrant humanity also includes one-eyed, four-eyed, eight-toed and twelve-fingered people, and some who use one ear as a bed sheet and the other as a blanket.

To do justice to the old chronicles, one must sort out their monsters into fact and fiction. Among the facts that time has vindicated stand out—to name a few—Licinius Mutianus' much challenged tale of having seen a boy changed into a girl; the unkissable lips of Chad women who, to this day, have suffered no loss of charm

89

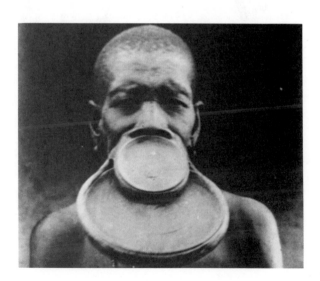

Chad woman.
(Courtesy, Musée de l'Homme, Paris)

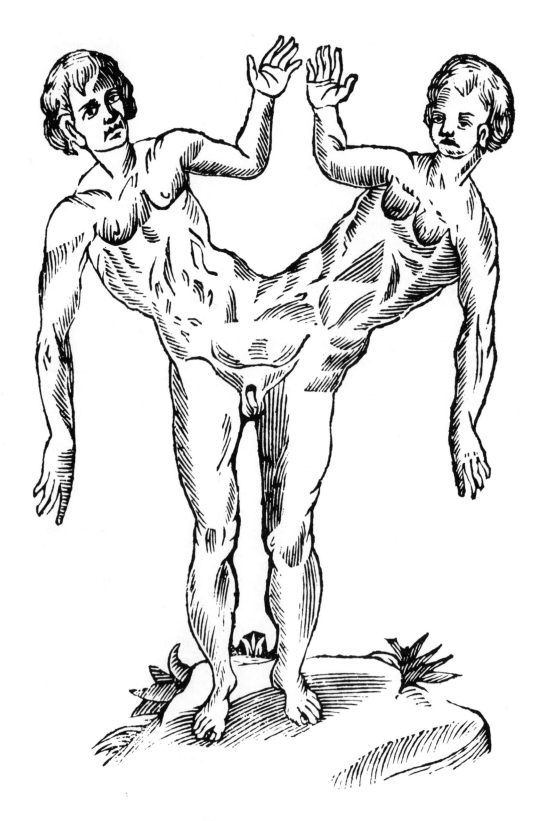

Malformation from Ulyssis Aldrovandi's
Monstrorum Historia, *1562.*

in the eyes of their lovers and husbands; humanoids with cyclop's eye or several eyes, several arms and legs, all known from teratology, a branch of embryology.

But mostly the public's fancy is caught by double and triple monsters, creatures welded together by an unkind fate. Despite their misfortune some of them lived to an old age, others attained fame for their special achievements. Perhaps best known are the Melionides, a pair joined together from the hips down, who fought Herakles with great aplomb. It seems that an uncommon sense of timing facilitates teamwork without curtailing the independence of each half of the binary being. Of so-called Siamese twins that lived during the reign of Emperor Theodosius it is reported that one head might be crying while the other was laughing, or one was eating while the other was sleeping.

Among these doubles who made news in more recent times were the Czech sisters Josepha and Rosa Blazek who were joined at the sacrum and part of the spinal column. The dissimilarity of their temperaments was best illustrated by their drinking habits. One had a preference for beer, the other for wine—a gulf wide enough to divide entire nations. However, we get an inkling of the complications attending an enforced dual life style only when we consider their case in the light of the causes and consequences of procreation. It is known that at the age of thirty-two the sisters entered a hospital in Prague where Rosa gave birth to a boy. Unfortunately, wedlock and domestic happiness were denied to her. The wedding never took place because the bridegroom would have been prosecuted for bigamy.

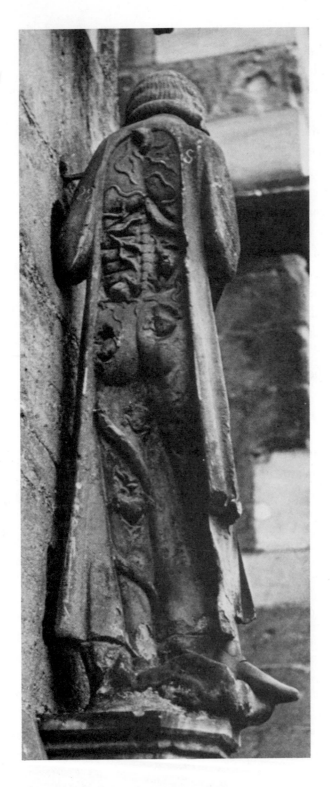

"Frau Welt." Rear view of a Gothic statue
outside of the Sebaldus Church in Nuremberg.
(Courtesy, Hauptamt für Hochbauwesen Nürnberg)

The fashionable body

The urge to alter his body is felt by man only; animals, enjoying
the advantage of healthier instincts, do not share it. Although the
human shape was designed by the greatest of artists, His taste does
not necessarily coincide with ours; at no time did man accept the
image in which he was created as final, and he early decided that
there was room for improvement. Neither prehistoric cave dweller
nor late-industrial urban man considered the human body aesthetically satisfactory; the Aurignacians and Magdalenians practiced mutilation of the hands with the same confidence that modern man
brings to crippling his feet. Uneducated and oversophisticated alike
seem to act on an uncontrollable impulse to rearrange their anatomy;
no part of the body is spared some more or less violent interference.
With all the points of similarity, however, there is one significant
difference: Primitive man sets up an unvarying body ideal and sticks
to it. Industrial man, on the other hand, has no clear idea of what he
wants; his aims are erratic, his tastes ephemeral. Whatever the reasons for wanting to change his physique, whatever the relevance of
his narcissistic or autoerotic inclinations, the factor that goes farthest
to account for this unholy obsession is his boredom. Bored with the
natural shape of his body, he delights in getting away from himself,

and to judge from past and present performances, the resources at hand for making his escape are inexhaustible. Not that there is much method in his endeavors; instead of striving for perfection he is consumed by a passion for unceasing experimentation. Only rarely does he exercise self-restraint. To the ancient Greeks, for instance, the human body was inviolate, or almost: they plucked their pubic hair. As a rule, however, man sees in his body little more than the raw material for his creations. The fact that his exertions can be traced back to prehistoric times does not sanction the results but endows them with a certain respectability.

In the beginning, man himself was clay and canvas. Body painting and body sculpture were fused into a single production and thus accounted for a harmonious work of art. Indeed, we should not hesitate to regard them as the oldest art. At any rate, the use of the body as the artist's medium rather than his inspiration antedates the more conventional categories of plastic art.[38]

Works of art often exist only in the minds of those who create them, and the so-called improvements perpetrated on our anatomy are no exception. "It is certainly not true," observed Charles Darwin, "that there is in the mind of man any universal standard of beauty with respect to the human body. It is, however, possible that certain tastes may in the course of time become inherited." Without going into the deeper motives of why certain human forms give us pleasure and others do not, Darwin scoffed at Western man's conceits. "If all our women," he argued, "were to become as beautiful as the Venus de' Medici, we should for a time be charmed; but we should soon wish for variety; and as soon as we had obtained variety, we should wish to see certain characteristics a little exaggerated beyond the then existing standards."[39] As we shall see, a little exaggeration goes a long way.

It is of course doubtful that a modern woman blessed with the proportions of a Greek statue would be happy. Broad hips have not been fashionable for a long time, and what modern shoe could accommodate a classical foot? But then, even in Darwin's time, the shape of the Medicean Venus (a mere copy of a Greek sculpture) was thought to be on the dowdy side. Far more desirable than everlasting perfection were, and still are, changeable beauty ideals, and with good reason:

Our laws permit a man to have as many wives as he pleases, provided he marries them successively. Since, however, this staggered sort of polygamy is often beyond a man's means, the way to make the monotony of marital life tolerable is to split a wife's personality. To appease her husband's promiscuous appetites, a good wife will impersonate as many divers types as her talents permit. Masquerading alone won't do the trick. A new dress or a sun tan do not turn her into a new woman; the change has to be more than skin-

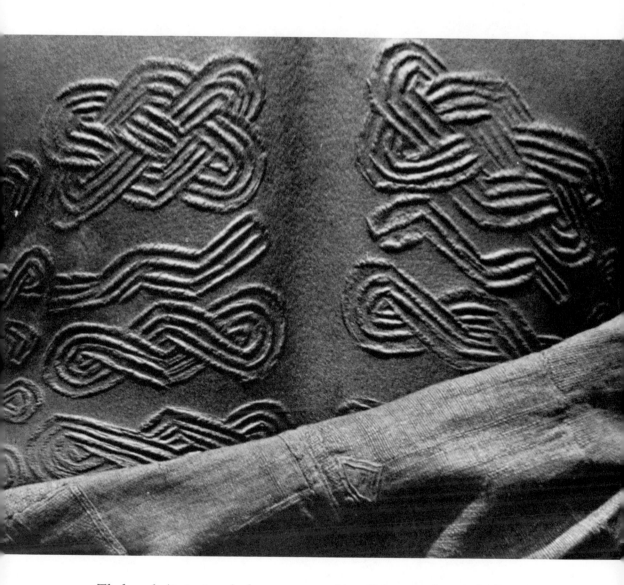

The bas-relief imitating a basket weave was achieved by cutting slits into the skin and rubbing charcoal or other foreign matter into them. The embossed epidermis thus becomes a keyboard for finger exercises; an audacious glissando may release sympathetic vibrations throughout the body. Bakuba tribe, Basongo, Congo. (Courtesy, Eliot Elisofon)

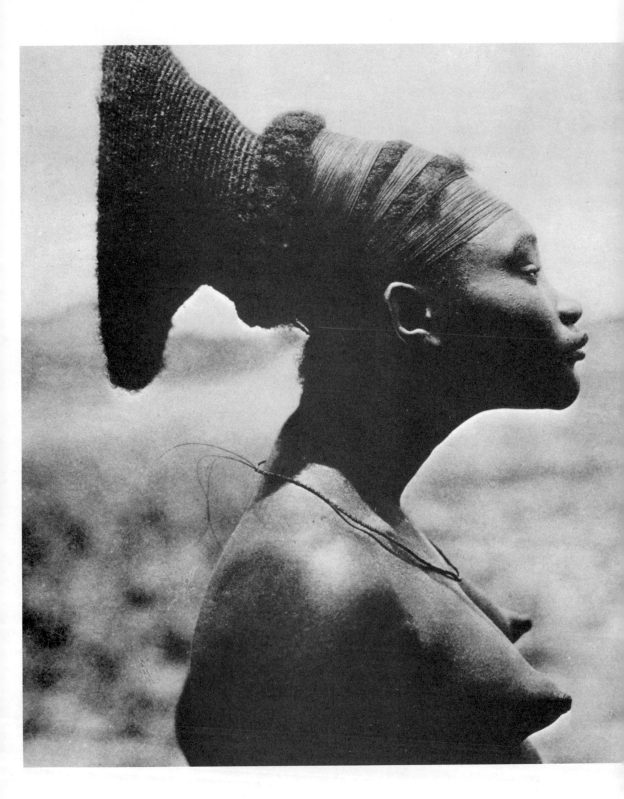

Mangbetu woman. Congo. (Courtesy, Musée de l'Homme, Paris)

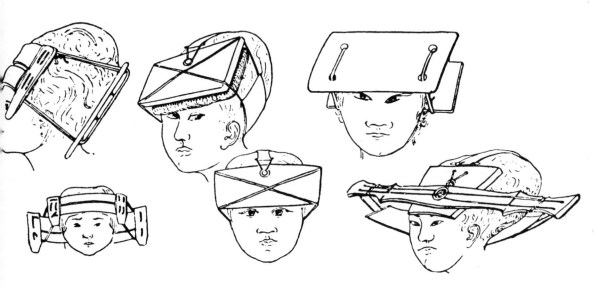

deep. In the following pages we shall examine, if ever so rapidly, some of the alterations that she—or he—were able to accomplish in their pursuit of physical variety. Let us begin at the top.

One of the boldest ways to interfere with human anatomy is the molding of the skull. Among tribes who practice this art, it is part and parcel of a child's upbringing. It calls for special skills and has traditionally been a mother's duty and, we may presume, pleasure. The first provocation to a mother's pinching and kneading her baby's skull was perhaps its yielding softness. Playful handling developed into more conscious efforts at deformation, to which racial and aesthetic concepts were added later. Thus, broad heads were broadened, flat noses flattened closer to the face, a tapering occiput sharpened to a point—a shape mostly associated today with humanoids from outer space. These spectacular forms were achieved with the aid of contraptions no more ingenious than a common mousetrap.

Admiration for elongated heads was widespread among such dissimilar peoples as the ancient Egyptians, American Indians, and provincial French. In some parts of France the custom of binding children's heads was still observed as late as the past century. Contrary to what one would expect from a nation known for setting ideals of elegance for the better part of the world, the motives for this kind of head deformation were eugenic rather than aesthetic. Educational systems being what they are, people believed that a child's vocation could be guided, literally, by shaping his brain. One Jesuit, Father Josset, for instance, advised mothers to work on their new-born children's heads so that they might become great orators.

It was a time when phrenology was the last word in head control. Purportedly a science, it dealt with the conformation of the skull. The shape of a person's head was supposed to determine his aptitudes and moral character. Indeed, it was thought that a direct relationship existed between the faculties of the mind and the separate portions of the brain, each portion representing a distinct mental or moral disposition. Their number varied from twenty-seven to thirty-six, depending on the phrenologist's persuasion. They were classified in what strike us today as rather whimsical categories: Religion; Wit; Ideality; Cunning; Marvellousness; Mimicry; Murder; Wonder; and so forth. Persons who had their heads examined

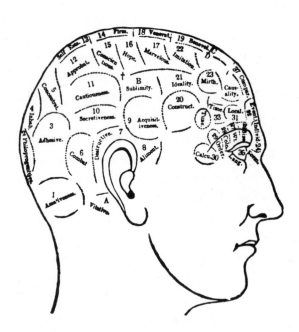

Phrenologists divided the surface of the brain into about three dozen regions which they identified as the seats of man's feelings and intellectual faculties. Diagram from the Phrenological Journal, 1842.

late in life often realized with dismay that they had missed a chance of being massaged into a genius. Eventually, the "art of reading bumps," as it was called in the United States, was so successful that an American university established a professorship of phrenology.[40] Observed the Encyclopaedia Americana: "The most necessary thing for a professor of phrenology was a happy faculty for flattering everybody."[41] Alas, not only art but also science is subject to the fashions of the day. Thus, phrenology has given way to aptitude tests, while squeezing heads has been abandoned in favor of squeezing toes.

Another, far more enduring, not to say endearing, sort of body deformation is obesity. Admired in many parts of the world, obesity rates—as far as women are concerned—as a secondary sexual characteristic. To judge from prehistoric art, fat women either predominated or were chosen by artists for their models, and in the course of time the well-upholstered woman was favored over the scrawny one. A similar taste can frequently be found in modern art; the artist who does not limit his sympathies to the fashionably disembodied female, sides with the primitive, and celebrates massive womanhood. Moreover, a fat body is often thought of as a strong body, and since only women of leisure can afford the luxury of being immobilized, the overfed woman came to represent the well-to-do and beautiful; obesity was promoted to a mark of quality. Hence among those primitives who gauge female beauty by sheer bulk, brides-to-be go through preparations of excessive fattening.[42] Upon reaching puberty, a girl is placed in a special fattening-house. The time of seclusion varies from several weeks to two years depending on the wealth of her parents.

Some tribes discriminate in their admiration for obesity between over-all bulk and specific, strategically placed cushions of fat. The most celebrated among salient features is steatopygia, the overdevelopment of the subcutaneous fat that covers a woman's hind parts and upper thighs. Unlike the judges of our beauty contests who have their eyes on a prominently cantilevered bosom, buttock lovers make their selection by "ranging their women in a line, and by picking *her* out who projects farthest *a tergo*."[43] Western woman, whom nature forgot to endow with a magnificent rear end, had at times to rely on make-believe to render herself desirable; witness the bustle of the eighteen-seventies, a gross illusion of steatopygia. Subsequently, man's admiration shifted to the stout woman with a tiny waist, a combination that does not occur in nature. It cannot be produced by crossbreeding or special exercise; it exists only as a sartorial illusion, achieved by applying a vise known as corset.

In approaching this subject we have to keep in mind that the

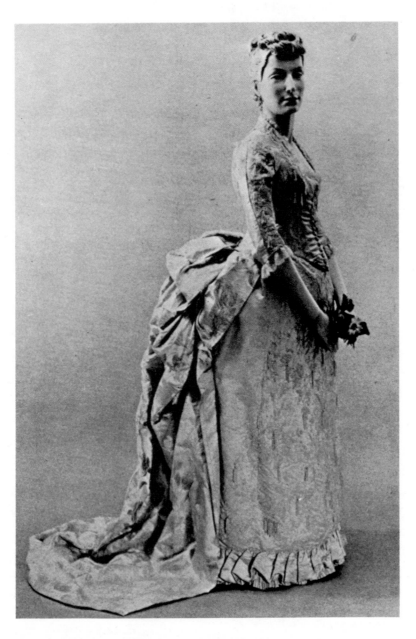

Three generations ago, steatopygia, whether genuine or simulated, was the rage of the day; "with many Hottentot women," wrote an enraptured Darwin, "the posterior part of the body projects in a wonderful manner."

woman who lived at the turn of the century barely resembled to-day's woman. She had missed an important phase in the evolution of mankind for she could not stand straight unaided. To insure her upright position she needed support, and it was the corset that saved her from having to walk on all fours.

Precautions against her breakdown had to be taken early in life. The little girl was securely encased in a junior corset that promised

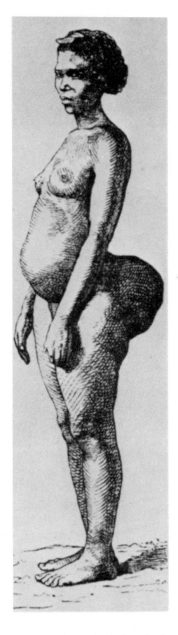

Opposite: American evening dress, c. 1885. (Courtesy, Museum of the City of New York)

Right: Gonaqua Hottentot from G.T. Fritsch, Die Eingeborenen Südafrikas.

If female dress were designed to follow a woman's contours, the bustle dress (opposite) would fit the Hottentot woman like a glove. Yet although the women's silhouettes are identical, the American's majestic posterior is but a sartorial illusion. (Courtesy, Museum of the City of New York)

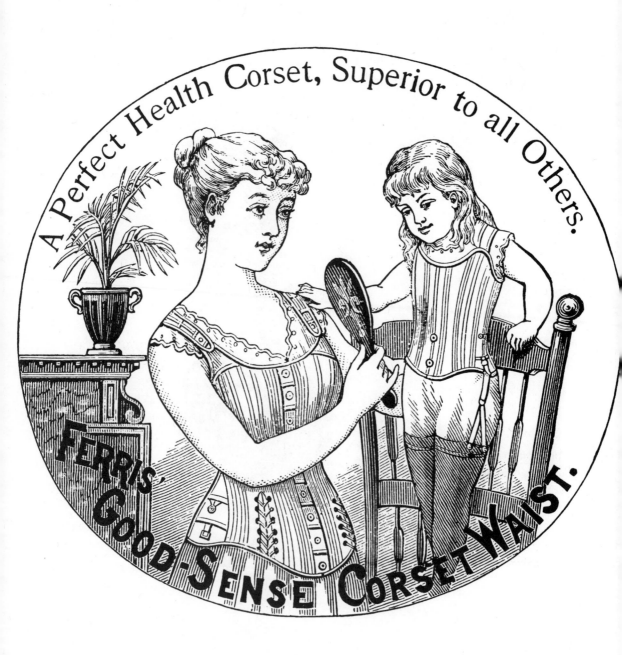

Advertisement from Harper's Bazar, *1886.*

Perfect Health, and visibly improved the contours of her shrimplike body. (To be sure, the use of a child's corset was not limited to occidental countries. Circassian girls—to give but one foreign example—wore from the tenth year on a broad girdle of untanned leather. The wealthy locked it with silver hooks whereas common people sewed it tightly around the waist. One writer, familiar with Circassian lore, tells us that mothers fastened their daughters "into saffian leather garments for seven years to give their figures symmetry."[44] This cuirass was worn until the wedding night "when the bridegroom with a sharp-cutting dagger unties the Gordian knot, which ceremony is frequently attended with danger.")[45]

The corset of our grandmothers was a masterpiece of functional design. It operated on three levels—mechanical, aesthetic, and moral. "The corset," wrote Thorstein Veblen, the foremost portraitist of the leisure class, "is in economic theory substantially [an instrument of] mutilation for the purpose of lowering the subject's vitality and rendering her personally and obviously unfit for work. It is true, the corset impairs the personal attractiveness of the wearer [Veblen refers of course to the naked woman], but the loss suffered on that score is offset by the gain in reputability which comes of her visibly increased expensiveness and infirmity."[46] The natural outline of the female waist, unredeemed by art, was not savory

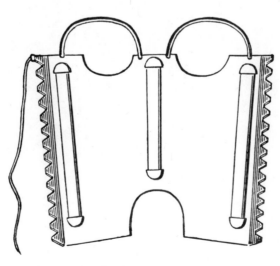

At the age of seven or eight, Ossetes girls (Central Caucasus) were clapped into this hard edge corset. From H. H. Ploss's Woman.

enough for man. It was the corsetière's business to attack the aesthetic problem at its roots by bending women's bones into an alluring shape.

The whalebone corset marked an advanced technique of disfigurement. Although the mechanism with its stays and ribbons was a comedown from the all-metal corset, the results were complex enough. Not only did the corset claw into the flesh, it played havoc with the inner organs by displacing them, eventually leading to a

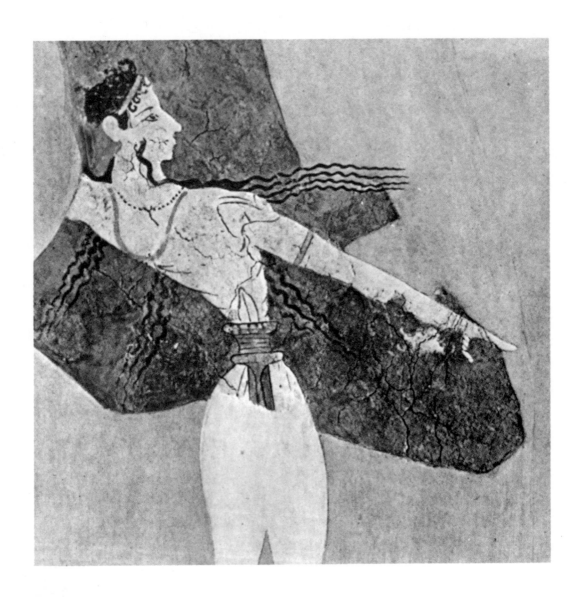

Fragmentary Minoan mural. Seventeenth or eighteenth century B.C.
From Sir Arthur Evans' The Palace of Minos at Knossos.

number of ailments. Occasionally, it caused miscarriages. On the credit side was the heightened seductiveness of the wearer, her embraceability, so to speak: the pressure applied to the waist produced the desired simultaneous inflation of the chest and buttocks, the latter still further accentuated by the bustle.

The corset's crippling effects on the female body were persistently ignored, much as today we ignore the consequences of wearing deforming shoes. The would-be guardian of our health, the physician,

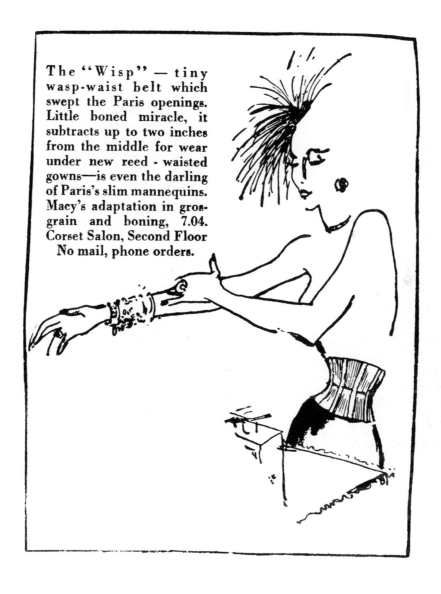

The "Wisp" — tiny wasp-waist belt which swept the Paris openings. Little boned miracle, it subtracts up to two inches from the middle for wear under new reed - waisted gowns—is even the darling of Paris's slim mannequins. Macy's adaptation in grosgrain and boning, 7.04. Corset Salon, Second Floor No mail, phone orders.

"Little boned miracle." Advertisement, 1946. (Courtesy of Macy's)

whose business it is to keep us in good working order, was then as reluctant to interfere with fashion's dictum as he is today. His warnings were sounded timidly, or at any rate ineffectively. He plied his trade oblivious of, or in tacit agreement with, the abuses of the day. As a man he was not immune to the corset's fascination; as a doctor he hesitated to condemn the corset for fear of being considered immoral. Respectful of manufacturers and their products, he did not permit himself much criticism. Occasionally, he was even known to pimp for them or, better, turn predatory and go into business himself.

To give an example—in the eighteen-eighties, a Dr. Scott put on the market an unbreakable electric corset, guaranteed quickly to

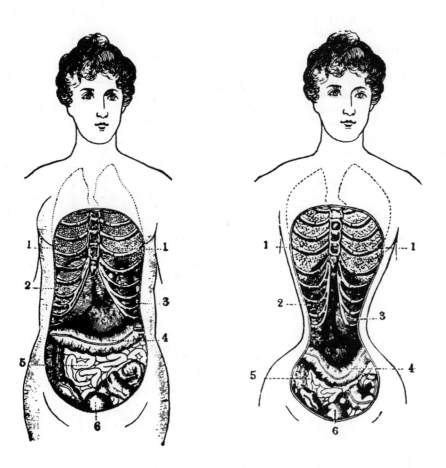

Effects of lacing on the female body. (*1 lungs, 2 liver, 3 stomach, 4 great-gut, 5 small intestine, 6 bladder*). *Nature, anticipating no doubt the invention of the corset, did not connect the lower five ribs to the breast bone. From* Reform-Moden-Album, *1904.*

1883---New Prices!---1883.
DR. SCOTT'S ELECTRIC CORSET.
$1, $1.50, $2, $2.50, $3.

Owing to the unprecedented success attending the sale and use of our $3 Electric Corset, and the constant demand for Electric Corsets of less price, but of the same therapeutic value, we have decided to place upon the market **A HANDSOME LINE OF ELECTRIC CORSETS**, ranging in price from $1 to $3, thus bringing them within the reach of all who desire them. They are equally charged with electro magnetism, the difference being only in the quality of material. The higher grades are made of extra fine English Sateen, while those of lesser price are of correspondingly good quality. All are made on the latest approved Parisian models, thus imparting a graceful and attractive figure to the wearer. By a recently invented process of boning or cording, we are enabled to offer to the public an **ABSOLUTELY UNBREAKABLE** Corset, and will guarantee them as such with all ordinary wear.

Being "**Electric**," "**Unbreakable**," the true French shape, and of **better material** than those ordinarily sold at the prices, these Corsets will command the preference of the purchaser. They are constructed on scientific principles, generating an exhilarating, health-giving current to the whole system. Their therapeutic value is unquestioned, and they quickly cure, in a marvelous manner, Nervous Debility, Spinal Complaints, Rheumatism, Paralysis, Numbness, Dyspepsia, Liver and Kidney troubles, Impaired Circulation, Constipation, and all other diseases peculiar to women, particularly those of sedentary habits. They also become, when constantly worn, equalizing agents in all cases of extreme fatness or leanness, by imparting to the system the required amount of "odic force" which Nature's law demands.

Scientists are daily making known to the world the indisputably beneficial effects of Electro-Magnetism, when properly and scientifically applied to the human body in this manner; and it is also affirmed by professional men that there is hardly a disease which Electricity and Magnetism will not benefit or cure, and all medical men daily practice the same. Ask your own physician!

DR. W. A. HAMMOND, of New York, Late Surgeon-General of the U. S., an eminent authority publishes almost miraculous cures coming under his notice. Always doing good, never harm, there is no shock or sensation felt in wearing them.

The ordinary Electric Battery, when resorted to in similar cases to those above mentioned, is often too powerful and exciting doing good during the operation, but leaving the patient more exhausted and weakened than before; whereas by daily (and nightly, too, if desired) wearing our Electric Corset as ordinary corsets are usually worn, a gentle and exhilarating influence is lastingly and agreeably perceptible, quickly accomplishing that good for which they are worn. They will never harm even in the most sensitive cases.

Ladies who have once tried them say they will wear no others. The prices are as follows: $1, $1.50, $2, $2.50 and $3. The two latter kinds are made in Pink, Blue, White and Dove; the others in White and Dove only. Each Corset is sent out in a handsome box, accompanied by a silver-plated compass, by which the electro-magnetic influence of the Corsets can be tested. We will send either kind to any address, postpaid, on receipt of the price; also add 10 cents for registration, to insure safe delivery. Remit in P. O. Money Order, Draft, Check, or in Currency, by Registered Letter.

In ordering, kindly **mention this publication,** and state exact size of Corset usually worn; or, where the size is not known, take a tight measurement of the waist over the linen. This can be done with a piece of common string, which send with your order. Make all remittances payable to

GEO. A. SCOTT, 842 Broadway, N. Y.

DR. SCOTT'S ELECTRIC HAIR BRUSH—new prices. $1, $1.50, $2, $2.50 and $3—sent postpaid on receipt of price.

PATENTED AND TRADEMARK ELECTRIC REGISTERED

N. B.—Each corset is stamped with the English coat-of-arms and the name PALL MALL ELECTRIC ASSOCIATION, LONDON.

SENT POST PAID ON TRIAL

The Electric Corset, an improvement over "those ordinarily sold," was a panacea against any number of diseases; it miraculously cured paralysis, dyspepsia, liver and kidney troubles. But only careful reading of the advertisement will disclose all its merits. From Harper's Bazar, 1883.

cure paralysis, rheumatism, spinal complaints, dyspepsia, constipation, impaired circulation, liver and kidney troubles, nervous debility, numbness, and so forth. "Constructed on scientific principles," the advertisement assured the gullible woman, "the therapeutic value is unquestioned." When constantly worn, "nightly, if desired," the corset also imparted to one's system "the required amount of *odic force* which Nature's law demands."

Odic force, a now forgotten nineteenth-century discovery, was then much on people's minds, thanks to the persuasive power of advertising. *Od* was a gift of nature, like perfect pitch. Those who had it were endowed with excruciating sensibility. They could divine a vein of ore in a mountain or, more spectacularly, start a pendulum swinging without touching it. Those whom nature had neglected could, if they wished, have recourse to odic contraptions such as Dr. Scott's corset whose miraculous powers were attested to, believe it or not, by the late surgeon general of the United States. Eventually, the scientific theory collapsed and *od* became odious.

Everything considered, doctors' knowledge of the female anatomy was less than perfect mainly because they based their observations on the deformed body. They were misinformed about such an elementary performance as breathing; not only woman's skeleton but also her breathing apparatus was thought to function differently from man's. "Until recent years," wrote Havelock Ellis in 1910, "it was commonly supposed that there is a real and fundamental difference in breathing between men and women, that women's breathing is thoracic and men's abdominal. It is now known that under natural and healthy conditions there is no difference, but men and women breathe in a precisely identical manner."[47] If doctors had wanted to they could easily have found "natural and healthy conditions" among non-corset-wearing women the world over.

Withal, corset manufacturers did not overlook the male body as potential modeling clay in their hands. Although the wearing of a corset was mainly a woman's prerogative (and duty), the fops and drones among men were not long in adopting it. "The corset mania," we read in the *Springfield Republican* of 1903, "began with the military men—they compare notes on corsets in some of the army clubs as gravely as they discuss the education bill at the National Library Club."[48] In all fairness, however, we must grant them in restrospect their inalienable right to body deformation. They were not the first to squeeze their waists; wasp waists were common as far back as archaic Greece. The last holdout for male waist constriction is Papua, provided the old customs are still honored.

At a distance of more than three generations, our great-grandmothers' fanatical loyalty to the wasp-waist ideal would seem absurd

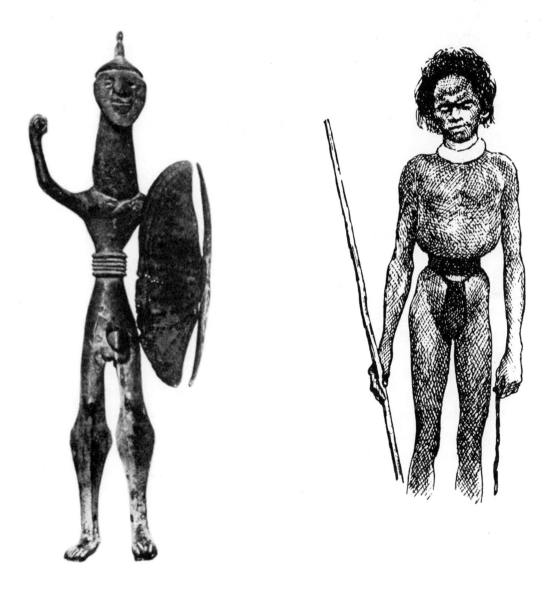

Left, archaic statuette with waist ring. National Museum, Athens.

Right, wasp-waisted Papuan. From Deformaciónes *by Dembo and Imbelloni.*

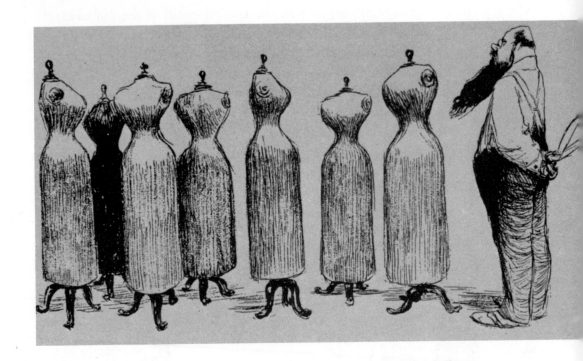

were it not that we now understand its deeper significance much better. Far more than a crutch, the corset was the hallmark of virtue. The belief that clothes are designed in good measure to punish the flesh never really lost its hold on us; in a way we are still doing penance for Adam's sin. Though clothes may not always be the best protection against nature's rigors, they often represent instruments of moral philosophy. The attraction of the agreeably punitive hairshirt has not worn off; metamorphosed variously into garter, girdle, waistband, and brassière, it plays on some of the focal points of the body, leaving an imprint. The bruises are accepted as the inevitable consequences of wearing clothes. Perhaps there lingers in women's mind the consoling thought that *their* mothers endured far greater inconvenience.

When the harm that resulted from wearing a corset had been belatedly recognized—and cavalierly dismissed—the fashion that lent an edge to men's inexhaustible appetite for swooning females was vindicated on moral grounds. People who lived in what was, from the point of view of costume history, a crustaceous age, thought of the whalebone corset as a kind of Jeanne d'Arc armor. Uncorseted women reeked of license; an unlaced waist was regarded as a vessel of sin. A heretic like Isadora Duncan, heralded by Rodin and other connoisseurs of the human physique as the embodiment of Greece, helped only to strengthen further the popular belief that the lack of a corset (and shoes) was the visible sign of depravity.

Every generation has its own demented ideas on supporting some part of the human anatomy. Older peole still remember a time when everybody went through life ankle-supported. Young and old wore laced boots. A shoe that did not reach well above the ankle was considered disastrous to health. What, one asks, has become of ankle support, once so warmly recommended by doctors and shoe salesmen? What keeps our ankles from breaking down these days of low-cut shoes?

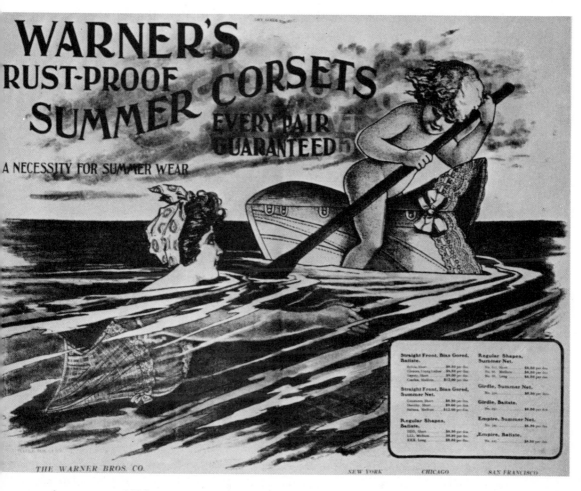

merican advertisement, 1901.

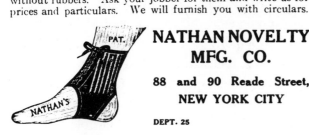
Advertisement for Ventilated Ankle Corset Support. 1883.

Ankle support has given way to arch support; millions of shoe-buying people are determined to "preserve their metatarsal arch" without as much as suspecting that it does not exist. Nevertheless, the fiction of the arch is being perpetuated to help sell "supports" and "preservers" on an impressive scale.

The dread of falling arches is, however, a picayune affair compared to that other calamity, the feet's asymmetry. I am not talking about the difference within a single pair of feet, that is, the difference between the right and left foot of a person; I mean the asymmetry of the foot itself.

Few of us are truly aware that an undeformed foot's outline is *not* symmetrical. It is distinctly lopsided. Let us have a close look at it: The big toe extends from one to two inches beyond the fifth toe. More importantly, the five toes spread out fanlike. They do not converge to a point in front as one would expect from the shape of the shoe. Quite the contrary, they converge to a point in back of the heel. It should be obvious, even to the least observant person, that to conform to the outline of a shoe, the big toe ought to be in the place of the third one, i.e. in the center.

Shoe manufacturers have shown admirable patience with nature. Despite or because of the absence of feet that live up to their commercial ideals of anatomy, they doggedly go on producing symmetrical shoes. And although their customers' feet have not changed in the course of time, they spare no effort and expense to come up every season with a new (symmetrical) shoe for the same old foot. (The pathological hate of the natural form of the foot is nowhere

The foot that fits the shoe: According to the gospel of our shoemakers, the big toe ought to be in the place of the third one. Hence shoes for symmetrical feet are not just a fashion but an unwritten law. To drive home the immensity of this abomination, Bernard Pfriem, portraitist of the human body par excellence, has obliged the author by interpreting the shoe designers' unfulfilled dream.

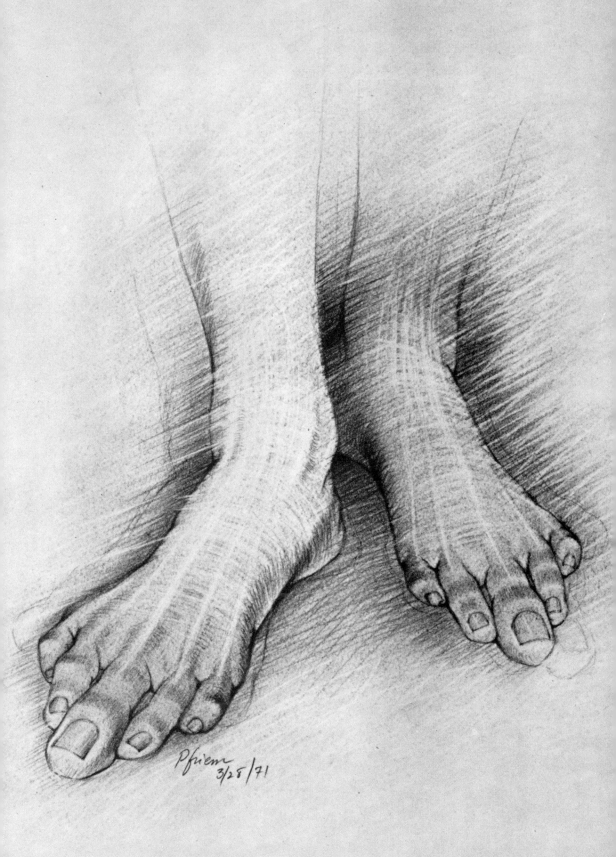

Pfriem
3/28/71

more forcibly expressed than in the commandments of the Shakers which say that "it is contrary to order to have right and left shoes.")

By some atavistic quirk of nature, every normal baby is born with undeformed feet. The forepart of the foot—measured across the toes—is about twice as wide as the heel. The toes barely touch each other and are as nimble as fingers. Were the child able to keep up his toe-twiddling, he might easily retain as much control over his feet as over his hands. Not that we see anything admirable in nimble toes; they strike us as freakish perhaps because we associate prehensile feet with primitive civilizations. To our twisted mind, the foot in its undamaged state is anachronistic, if not altogether barbaric. Ever since the shoe became the badge of admission to Western civilization—in rural countries such as Portugal and Brazil the government exhorts peasants to wear shoes in the name of progress—we look down on barefooted or sandaled nations.

Since wearing shoes is synonymous with wearing *bad* shoes, the modern shoe inevitably becomes an instrument of deformation. The very concept of the modern shoe does not admit of an intelligent solution; it is not made to fit a human foot but to fit a wooden last whose shape is determined by the whims of the "designer." Whereas a tailor allows for a customer's unequal shoulders and arms; an optometrist prescribes different lenses for the right and left eye, we

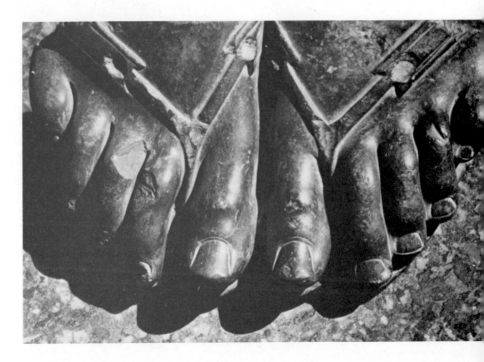

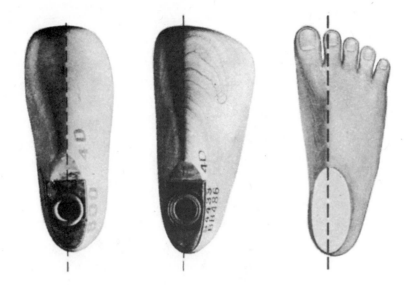

buy shoes of identical size and dimensions for our right and left foot, conveniently forgetting—or ignoring—that, as a rule, they are not of the same width and length. Even in countries where it is still possible to find an artisan willing to make a pair of shoes to order, chances are that he works on mass-produced lasts and comes up with a product that, shapewise, is not much different from the industrial one.

In both the manufacturer's and the customer's opinion the shoe comes before the foot. It is less intended to protect the foot from cold and dirt than to mold it into a fashionable shape. Infants' very first shoes are liable to dislocate the bones, and bend the foot into the shoe shape. The child does not mind the interference; "never expect the child to complain that the shoe is hurting him," says podiatrist Dr. Simon Wikler, "for the crippling process is painless." According to a ten-year study of the Podiatry Society of the State of New York, 99 percent of all feet are perfect at birth, 8 percent have developed troubles at one year, 41 percent at the age of five, and 80 percent at twenty; "we limp into adulthood," the report concludes. "Medical schools," says Dr. DePalma, "fail almost completely in giving the student a sound grounding and a sane therapeutic concept of foot conditions." And in *Military Medicine* one reads that "there has been no objective test that could be readily incorporated

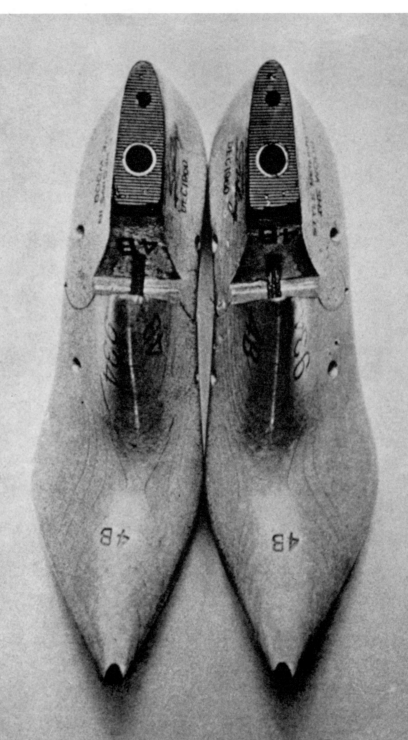

I. Miller builds a shoe
(and new shapes begin first with the Last)

in physical examinations, or taught to medical students, pediatricians, or physicians in military and industrial medicine, that would enable them to recognize deformities of the foot . . . "[49] In sum, physicians leave it to the shoe designer to decide the fate of our feet.

To top it all, modern man, perhaps unknown to himself, is afflicted with a diffuse shoe-fetishism. Inherited prejudices derived from the Cinderella complex; practices whose origins and reasons escape him, and traditional obtuseness combine to make him tolerate the deformities inflicted by his shoes. In this respect his callousness matches that of the Chinese of old. In fact, if he ever felt a need to justify the shoes' encroachments on his anatomy, he could cite Lily feet (provided he had ever heard of them), the Chinese variety of the "correctly shaped" foot.

This exotic custom which lasted nearly one thousand years did not extend over the whole country; the Manchu, including the imperial family, never practiced foot-binding. Small feet are a racial characteristic of Chinese women, and the desire to still further reduce their size in the name of beauty and for reasons indicated earlier, seems to have been strong enough to make women tolerate irrevocable mutilation. As so often happens, people derive infinitely greater satisfaction from an artifact, however crude, than from nature's product. Besides, not only were a woman's stunted feet

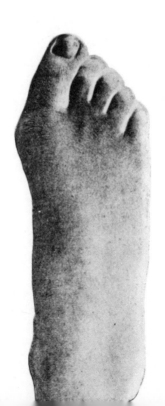

Adult foot, deformed from wearing conventional shoes.

highly charged with erotic symbolism, they made her eligible for marriage. Without them she was reduced to spinsterhood.[50] Her desirability as a love object was in direct proportion to her inability to walk. It ought to be easy for our women to understand the Chinese men's mentality; "every woman knows that to wear 'walking shoes'—as derogatory a term as 'sensible shoes'—puts a damper on a man's ardor. The effect of absurdly impractical shoes, on the other hand, is as intoxicating as a love potion. The girl child who puts on a pair of high-heeled shoes is magically propelled into womanhood."[51]

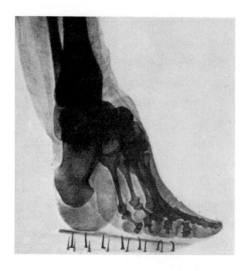

X-ray picture of a Chinese
woman's deformed foot.
Zeitschrift für Ethnologie, 1903.

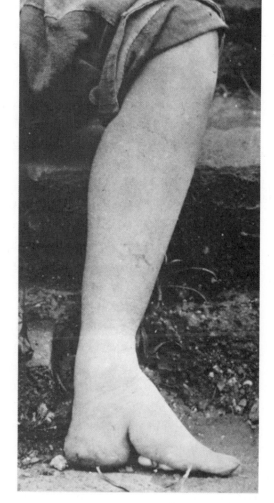

The organically grown high heel of Chinese women
anticipated modern woman's artificial heel.
(Courtesy, Musée de l'Homme, Paris)

While the custom of shaping women's feet according to a national ideal has long been
outlawed by the Chinese, Western man and woman have not outgrown their infatuation
with the symmetrical foot. (Courtesy, Musée de l'Homme, Paris)

Modern woman is not averse to maltreating her feet for reasons similar to those of her Chinese sisters, and therefore makes allowance for bunions, calluses, corns, ingrown toenails and hammer toes. But she draws the line at a major interference with her foot skeleton. Unwilling to bother with growing her own, organic high heels, she has to get along with artificial ones.

As costume props go, the high heel's history is relatively short. In the middle of the seventeenth century this new device for corrupting the human walk was added to the footwear of the elegant, putting them, as it were, on tiptoe. The ground, indoors and outdoors, came to a tilt, so to speak, and, for fashion's sake, people began to walk on a portable incline. As the ordinary folk continued to wear flat-bottomed shoes, heeled footwear, combined with a strutting walk, became a mark of distinction. Withal, the times were anything but favorable to the new invention. On the street the well-heeled had to avail themselves of a sedan chair to avoid the cobblestones underfoot, while indoors they found it difficult to negotiate the polished parquets and marble floors that were the pride of the epoch. And yet, men took to high heels as enthusiastically as women did. To judge from paintings of the time, fashionable men could not have cared less for "walking shoes."

Did men's high-heeled shoes and fine stockings turn a woman's head? Were women smitten with the sight of a man's well-turned ankle and slender leg? For whereas their own legs remained hidden by crinolines, men proudly displayed their calves and gave as much attention to them as to their wigs. Silicon injections still being centuries away, a skinny fellow made up by padding for any natural deficiency. Eventually, the French Revolution brought men and women down to earth. Dandies and *élégantes* wore paper-thin flat soles without, it seems, depriving themselves of their mutual attraction. Years later, when high heels reappeared on the fashionable scene, they were relegated to woman's domain; men never left the ground again.

In lucid moments we look with amazement at the fraud we perpetrate on ourselves—the bruises, mutilations, and dislocated bones —but if we feel at all uncomfortable, it is not for long. An automatic self-defense mechanism blurs our judgment, and makes right and wrong exchange places. Moreover, some violations of the body are sanctioned by religion, while others are simply the price of a man's admittance to his tribe, regardless of whether he lives in the bush or in a modern metropolis. The sense of superiority he derives from, say, circumcision is no less real than that of the owner of a pair of Lily feet. Physicians have always been of two minds about it; "to cut off the top of the uppermost skin of the secret parts," maintained the intrepid Dr. Bulwer, "is directly against the honesty of nature, and an injurious unsufferable trick put upon her."[52] And a contemporary pediatrician, E. Noel Preston, writing in the *Journal of the American Medical Association*, considers circumcision "little better than mutilation." The very real dangers of the operation such as infection and hemorrhage outweigh the fancied advantages of cancer prevention. "If a child can be taught to tie his shoes or brush his teeth or wash behind the ears," said Dr. Preston, "he can also be taught to wash beneath his foreskin."

A change of allegiance may lead to double mutilation, as in the paradoxical phenomenon of uncircumcision: After the subjugation of Palestine by Alexander the Great, those Jews who found it desirable to turn into Gentiles, underwent a painful operation that restored to them the missing prepuce. (1 Cor. 7:18 ff; 1 Macc. 1:15)

Sometimes such mutilation reaches a high degree of ferocity. Among some Arabian tribes circumcision is performed as an endurance test for youths who have come of age; "it consists," writes the Hebrew scholar Raphael Patai, "in cutting off the skin across the stomach below the navel and thence down the thighs, after which it is peeled off, leaving the stomach, the pelvis, the scrotum, and the inner legs uncovered and flayed. Many young men are said to have succumbed to the ordeal which in recent times has been prohibited by the Saudi Arabian government."[53] However, the custom has not disappeared, doubtless as a result of its sex appeal. The ceremony takes place in female company, that is, in the presence of the young men's brides-to-be, who may refuse to marry their intended if they betray their agony by as much as an air of discomfort.

Man's obsession with violating his body is not just of anthropological interest, it helps us to understand the irrationality of dress.

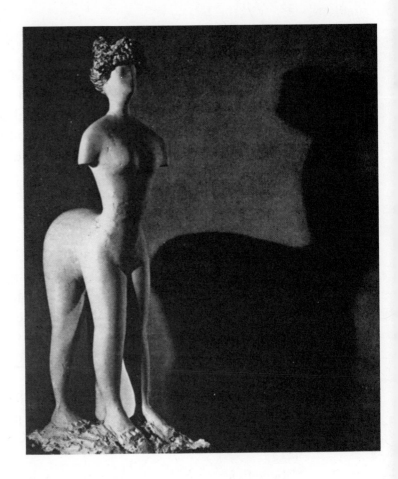

From time to time, the female figure is being revamped, much like automobile bodies or shop fronts. The four plaster figures, designed by the author and modeled by Costantino Nivola, show the shape of a woman's body as it might have looked had it corresponded to the shape of clothes in four different periods: 1. A woman of the eighteen seventies whose figure literally conformed to the bustle. 2. The dowager type with the shelf-like, cantilevered monobosom of 1904. 3. The hobbleskirted woman of 1913 who seemed to have a single leg. 4. The concave flapper of the nineteen-twenties. From the author's 1944 exhibition "Are Clothes Modern?" at the Museum of Modern Art, New York.

The devices for interfering with human anatomy are paralleled by a host of contraptions that simulate deformation or are simply meant to cheat the eye: bustles, pads, heels, wedges, braguettes, brassières, and so forth. Once, thirty years marked the end of a woman's desirability. In time, this age limit was gradually extended and pushed to a point where it got lost altogether. In order not only to look eternally young but also fashionable, woman had to obey ever-changing body ideals. Thus a woman born at the turn of the century was a buxom maiden in accordance with the dictates of the day. Photographs testify to the generosity of her charms although her tender age ought to raise doubts about their authenticity. In the nineteen-twenties, when maturity and motherhood had come to her, pictures record an angular, lean, flat-chested creature. Since she did not want to renounce her attractiveness, she had to submit

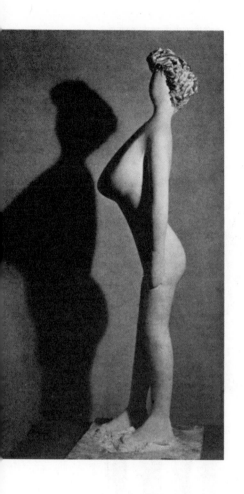 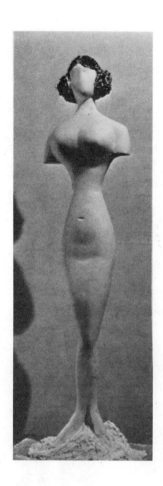 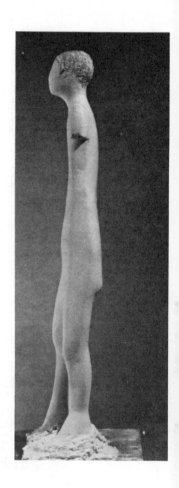

to an extremely unfeminine beauty ideal. Twenty years later, she was rotund again and commanded the undiminished attention of the other sex. Today, she is still in the running, ever ready to overhaul her body to prolong her youth beyond biological limits. She has inflamed three generations of men each loyal to a different image of perfection.

Alas, an aged body, however arresting and deceptive be the results of its updating and remodeling, imparts to its owner only a limited sense of youth. It serves mainly as a stylish peg for clothes. In other words, it is the clothed body that triumphs, not the naked one. As Herbert Spencer said: "The consciousness of being perfectly dressed may bestow a peace such as religion cannot give."

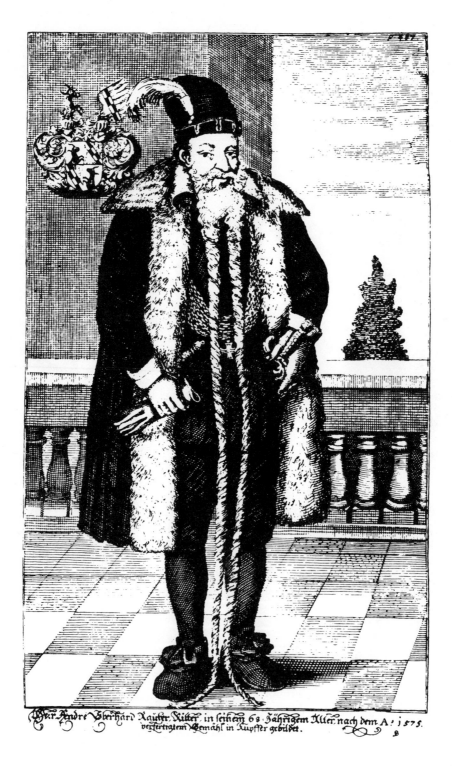

André Eberhard Raucher, a son-in-law of Emperor Maximilian II, cultivated a beard of such length that it gently swept the ground in front of him. Sixteenth-century engraving. (Courtesy, Picture Collection, New York Public Library)

The decorative arts

When man emerged from the ravages of evolution, he had forfeited
a number of features that once had stood him in good stead. Gone
was his tail. So was the prehensibility of his feet; the toes simply
lost their grip when he descended from his original habitat, the
trees. He could not wriggle his ears any more nor twitch his skin
although this was of lesser consequence. By far the greatest loss
was his thick coat of hair. Today he shares the nakedness of his
skin with the hippopotamus, elephant, and whale, none of them
particularly attractive creatures. All that is left of his hirsuteness
are some islands of straggling hair; a few tufts and ringlets—mere
vestiges of his former splendor—adorn his chest and, if he is lucky,
his arms and legs. Fads and fashions apart, his most precious growth,
face hair, lies fallow.

There is little doubt that abundant facial hair bestows authority
on man; a clean-shaven patriarch cuts a poor figure whereas a
bearded one invites confidence by milking his beard as if it were
an udder brimming with wisdom. The very act of stroking it adds
weight to his pronouncements. A beard commands respect; indeed,
it is the very symbol of respectability. The images of God the
Father and the prophets—including Mohammed and Freud—are

unthinkable without beards. So are alien gods and the heroes of epic poems. Zeus and Wotan, King Arthur and Charlemagne, wore free-flowing beards, while Hercules was celebrated for his hairy nates. More significantly, our first father, Adam, was created with a full-grown instant beard. Old civilizations held the beard sacred. Men swore by it. To pull a man's beard, or to cut it off, were deadly insults. The hairy bib, especially a blond one, radiated, if not sanctity, at least the sanctimoniousness of an upside-down halo.

A beard also symbolized virility. "The beard may be regarded as purely sexual ornament," wrote Havelock Ellis, himself a veritable bird of paradise among bearded men; "its history is interesting, for it illustrates the tendency with the increase of civilization not merely to dispense with sexual allurement, but even to disregard these growths which would appear to have developed solely to act as sexual allurements."[54] Which is to say that the man who shaves is the poorer for it.

Not only was the possession of a luxuriant beard a matter of pride to man in times past, its cultivation and care were considered agreeable duties. Besides, the hairdresser's repertory was incomparably more versatile than it is today. Five thousand years ago, a fastidious man had his beard dyed, oiled, and scented. It was pleated, curled, frizzled or starched, as can be plainly verified from fashion plates cut in stone. A Persian gentleman of high rank, availing himself of special barbershop privileges, might have his beard powdered with gold dust, or shot through with gold thread. It is well to keep in mind that such beard fashions were not mere episodes in costume history but lasted fifteen centuries.

Scarcely less arresting, though admittedly somewhat ambiguous, are female beards. The bearded woman of the fair booth is not unprecedented in history and neither is the use of false hairpieces. The Sumerian Great Mother Ivanna was shown with a beard, and Cypriotes worshiped a bearded Aphrodite, symbol of luxuriant growth and productivity. (Not to be outdone, Christian martyrology boasts of a bearded female saint, Wilgefortis—*virgo fortis*—a virgin who met death by crucifixion.) The full regalia of a Persian queen occasionally included a beard, a postiche held in place by a golden chin strap. Women with false beards are represented on Greek vases, and in Argos, Plutarch tells us, brides sleeping with their husbands for the first time, wore false beards to deceive the demons.

Through the centuries, beards and non-beards existed side by side. Hairstyles changed but not the arguments for and against them. Partisans constituted not just dandies and barbers but sometimes philosophers. Schopenhauer, for example, considered beards abominable. "Just look," he complained, "at the profile of a beard-man while he eats!"[55] To wear a sexual characteristic right in the middle of his face ("*mitten im Gesicht*") was, as he said, obscene. To his mind, a beard brutalized a man's face; the lifeless mass of hair covers, as he put it, exactly that part of the face "which expresses morality."[56] A vociferous advocate of shaving, he argued that a beard masked the face and thereby protected the criminal. Beards, he said, ought to be forbidden by law.

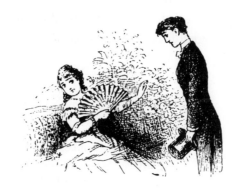

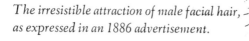

The irresistible attraction of male facial hair, as expressed in an 1886 advertisement.

One has to go back to the Elizabethans to find a spirited defender of beards and long hair. In his *Man Transform'd, or The Artificial Changeling*, John Bulwer wrote: "That hair should be a most abject excrement, an unprofitable burden, and a most unnecessary and uncomely covering, and that nature did never intend that excrement for an ornament, is a piece of ignorance or rather malicious impiety against nature."[57] His opinion was not shared by his compatriots this side of the Atlantic where, then as now, adults and adolescents who indulge in non-accredited hairstyles risk ostracism. Today, as in the past, the length of hair is a subject of debate.

The Harvard College Book of 1649 decreed: "For as much as the wearing of long hair after the manner of ruffians and barbarous Indians has begun to invade New England and contrary to the rule of God's word which says it is a shame for a man to wear long hair." The spirit of this ordinance still survives in the thirteen original states. In 1966, students in the State of Virginia petitioned the Supreme Court in vain to revoke an order of their school that made the orthodox American haircut a condition for their admittance. A Connecticut high school suspended fifty-three boys because "their

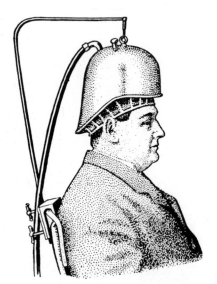

Opposite: As a symbol of authority, the wig ranks only slightly below that other exalted head ornament, the nimbus. The bust portrays the pleasure-loving Giovan Gastone, last duke of the Medici. The avalanche of ringlets has lost none of its delicate quality by being translated into marble.

A Scientific Method of Growing Hair

Advertisement, 1910.

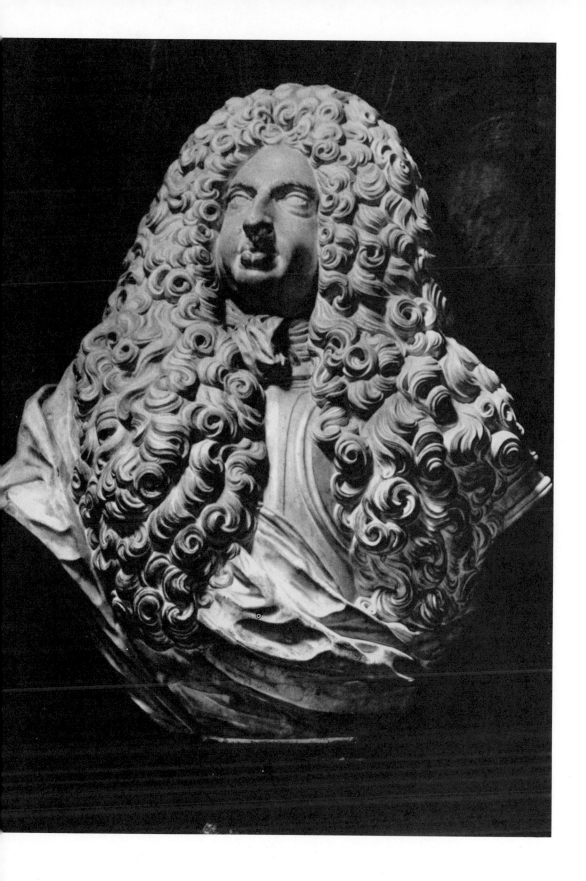

hair fashions detract from the healthy atmosphere conducive to good educational practice." In Philadelphia, high school students were required to shave off their mustaches or face suspension—a plain case of symbolic castration. And in New York State, a number of young martyrs in the cause of hirsuteness were deprived of their right to attend school; others were isolated from their fellow students by being placed—for lack of an old-fashioned pillory—at a penitential desk. Not until the American Civil Liberties Union came to the boys' rescue were the schoolmasters put in their place.

Soon the war against hair spread to Europe. In the spring of 1967, an announcement issued by the Ministries of Interior and Public Order in Athens barred foreign tourists with beards or long hair from visiting Greece. If the bearded or long-haired male insisted on entering the country, the announcement continued, "he must cut off his hair and beard and not grow them again." The order, commented the *New York Times*, was based on "a vision of a Greece returned to the practice of Spartan virtues and of Christian religion." It did not say whether the suppression of male hair growth applied retroactively to Spartan heroes and Christian saints.

It is of course known that Alexander the Great established a sort of precedent in these matters when he ordered his soldiers to shave their chins. The reason was plain for all to see, for a beard was truly a liability in those days. In hand-to-hand combat the adversary would grab it and hold on to it, much as fighting turkey cocks

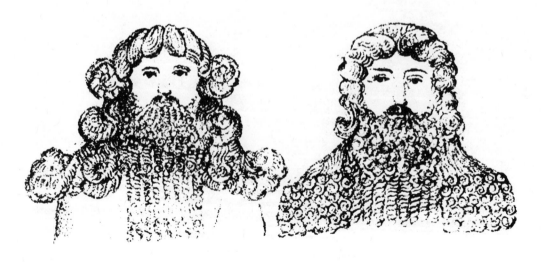

Although a luxuriant growth of male hair is again accepted in our society, its practical application has been overlooked so far. The picture suggests possibilities of how to convert live hair into scapularies and sweaters.

Vegetable fibers braided into the women's hair constitute veritable cloaks for a chieftain's wives. New Guinea. (Courtesy, Musée de l'Homme, Paris)

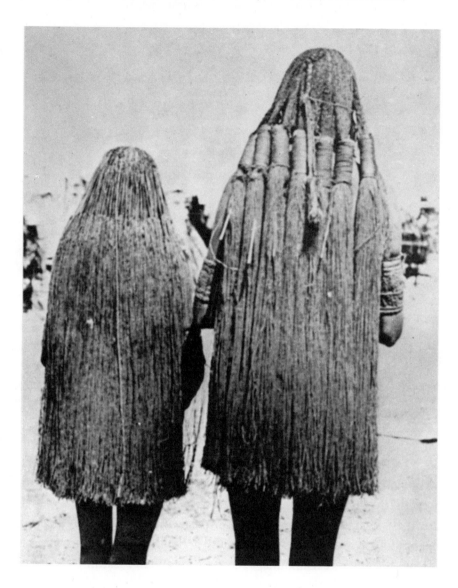

seize each others' wattles.

A society that penalizes nonconformity and the expression of the individual generates hairdressing problems also for its civil servants. In 1965, the New York Transit Authority ruled that no employee who comes into direct contact with the public should be allowed to wear a beard because "a beard on a [subway] platform tends to scare children and provoke compaints from mothers."[58] Whatever the motives of the beard haters, the very idea that American children

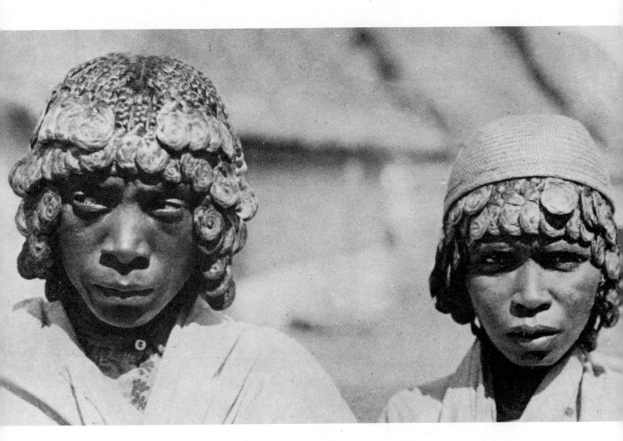

are afraid of beards is patently absurd. Whoever has watched them snuggle up to Santa Claus can attest to the irresistible *appeal* of his beard. It is precisely the tousled hairpiece in which the child puts his trust. God only knows what kind of fellow may be hiding behind it, yet his holiday camouflage confers temporary sainthood upon him.

On the whole, long hair and beards are not worn so much for looks as in protest against a society grown fat on prejudice. Besides, the crew cut, one of the least flattering hairstyles in history, is still favored by the conformist. It hardly is an advance over the convict's clean-shaven head, and few cases are known where it improved a man's physiognomy. But such is not its purpose; on the contrary, it is meant to deflect attention from the surface to the inner man. A kind of sawed-off nimbus, the crew cut carries a message that a fellow crew cut cannot miss.

Though both sexes have made use of false hairpieces all along, men have not yet taken to wearing false eyelashes; their use is restricted to Western and Westernized woman. Curiously, many races prefer the naked, unciliated eye, and pluck their brows and lashes as well as all other facial hair. In the Trobriands, an island group in New Guinea, the nibbling of eyelashes plays a part in love-making. "I have not seen," writes ethnographer Bronislav Malinowski, "one boy or girl in the Trobriands with the long lashes to which they are entitled by nature."[59] The reason for this, he explains, is that ardent lovers (and such they would seem to be) bite off each other's lashes at the height of ecstasy. The result are naked eyelids which enhance a person's amatory status. Whatever its merits, this symbolic devouring is unknown among us; besides, it is not recommended since one would risk ending up with a mouthful of the artificial stuff.

Eyebrows, too, are not always rated an asset, at least not in their natural state. The fear that a familiar face breeds boredom made women follow eyebrow fashions as transitory as lip fashions. For variety's sake they have been wearing their brows thin or thick, light or dark, long or short, arched or straight, and when they had exhausted all variations they removed them altogether. An example in point are the Japanese ladies of the Heian period (794–1185). Contemporary paintings show them with their eyebrows completely shaved off, their faces painted a ghostly white. The brows reappear, bigger and better, several inches higher, brushed in black on their

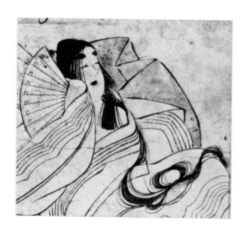

Ten centuries ago Japanese ladies wore permanently raised eyebrows. Detail from a scroll of the Kamakura Period. (Courtesy, Spencer Collection, New York Public Library)

forehead, lending the face a permanent expression, half quizzical, half haughty.

Man's inferiority vis-à-vis the animals becomes apparent when we examine the *hairless* areas of his skin. Although one may be of two minds about it, there is no denying that a fair complexion is a negative characteristic, denoting a scant supply of pigment. Having been left out of Nature's color scheme, White Man tries to attach aesthetic values to pallor and declares his skin color to be the very mark of superiority. Such sophistry is unconvincing for is not a bronzed skin more attractive than a pale one? If it is not, why do we bother with baking in the sun or under a sun lamp to get a tan? Indeed, why is the albino not king among us? A tanned person looks better or at least healthier than an untanned one even though the tan most likely is mere patchwork. Instead of spreading over the body's entire surface, it stops short of the intimate parts which, modesty decrees, must be covered even when sea- or sunbathing. The result is a ribald pattern, as weird as war paint.

When it comes to body painting proper, primitive peoples often abandon all pretense to imitating flesh tones, as did, for example, Britain's aborigines who resolutely painted, or tattooed, their bodies blue. Both so-called savages and civilized people seem to take exception to a blank body even though their ideas about improving its appearance may differ widely. By and large, primitive man is the more imaginative of the two. He often covers the entire body with paint, making it look fully dressed. Free as he is of our conventions of modesty and fashion, he gets his painterly inspiration from the kaleidoscopic hues of his immediate environment, more especially from animals. The adult mandrill, a member of the baboon family, has the ancient Briton's blue face, plus a two-tone blue-and-red behind. The colors are not lost on the beasts. Half-wild horses are attracted by those of the same coloring, and so are fallow deer. More surprisingly, some animals can be duped by the art of make-up. "A female zebra," noted Darwin, "would not admit the addresses of a male ass until he was painted so as to resemble a zebra, and then she received him very readily."[60] It stands to reason that man's desire to paint and ornament his body goes beyond a craving for beauty; coloration and ornament are chiefly stimulants to sexual

Maquillage by Saul Steinberg.

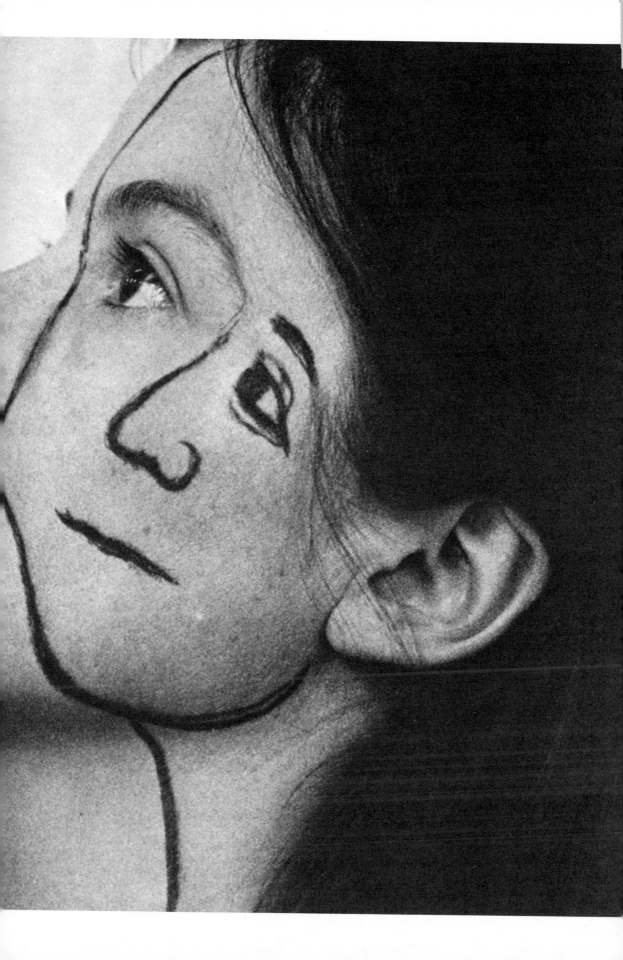

selection. Among underdressed African tribes where men rather than women go in for elaborate decorations, spinsters are unknown; celibacy is confined to men.

At present, modern man is not permitted to paint himself freely. Should he want to radiate manliness he has to take recourse to pills and lotions or the time-consuming process of tanning. Neither does woman indulge in body painting. She is perfectly satisfied with painting her face, spreading the cosmetic pigment over an area bordered by the roots of her hair and the base of her neck. The

136

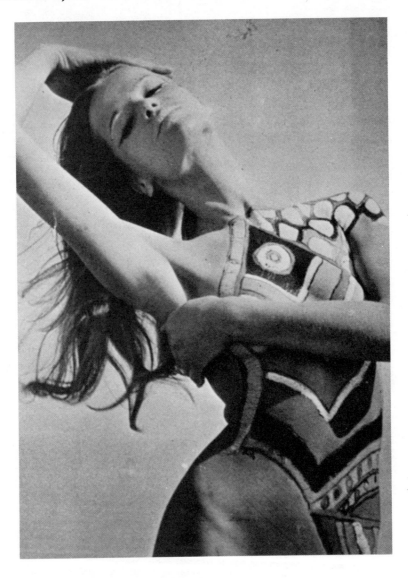

Paint, simulating a garment. (Courtesy, Vogue.
Copyright © 1966 by The Condé Nast Publications, Inc.)

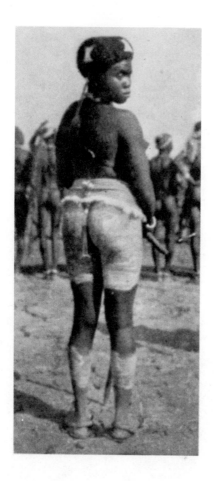

Body painting, inspired by British officers' shorts.

more fastidious among them may rouge lobules and nipples, perhaps knee caps and elbow tips, in imitation of past practices. Occasionally, an elegant woman's magazine will tease the reader with visions of transcendent beauty by showing a woman's belly decorated with an abstract painting yet this abdominal work of art looks curiously tame. Far from conjuring up cannibals, it calls circus people to mind.

The earliest instance of American body painting on record is that of a young woman from Arkansas who "desirous of making a brilliant figure at a ball, called a paintbrush and a quantity of red and white paint to her aid, and produced on those present at the ball the impression that she was wearing a beautiful and costly pair of striped stockings." It happened in 1879, and was duly reported in the *New York Times*.

One century later, the painted stocking is still the only instance of Western body art that simulates apparel. Much in vogue hereabouts in the nineteen-forties, it was characterized by crude coloring matter that came off on upholstery, clothes, and fellow creatures. Unlike nylon stockings, however, it did not disintegrate in our cities' poisonous atmosphere. A revival of leg painting, staged twenty years later, departed from flesh tones and thus set the scene for more ambitious exploits.

Body painting may not be much distinguished for refinement but tattooing certainly is—always excepting our kind of parlor-tattooing. The difference between the unrestricted body painting and tattooing of primitive peoples and our own timid ventures is about the same

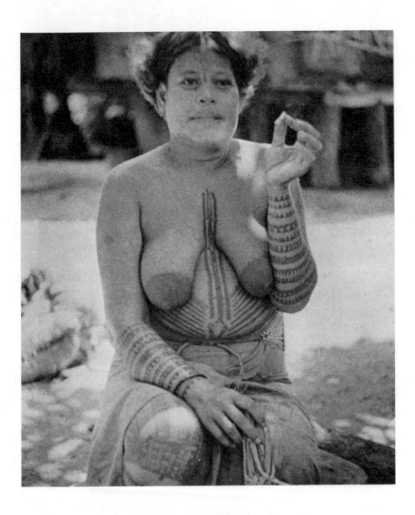

Tattoo. Ontong. Java Island. (Courtesy, Eliot Elisofon)

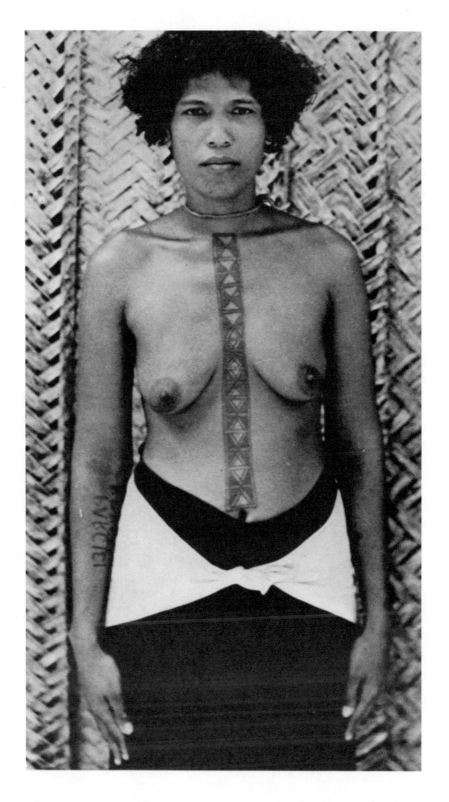

There is nothing primitive or inelegant about this woman's get-up. Neckring, skirt, and the severe abstraction of a blouse add up to what can only be called a festive outfit. Stewart Island. (Courtesy, Musée de l'Homme, Paris)

as that between a decorated Russian Easter egg and a plain egg. To a painter, one would think, the human body presents a far more enticing surface than flat canvas or a wall, though in practice it does not. Nearly a century ago, Alexander von Humboldt pointed out that body painting is nowise inferior to the art of dress. "If painted nations," he wrote, "had been examined with the same attention as clothed ones, it would have been perceived that the most fertile imagination and the most mutable caprice have created the fashions of painting as well as those of garments."[61] A good many examples

Anthropologists have ascertained that no part of the body is safe from tattooing. People are known to have tattooed their lips, gums, genitals, even the tip of the tongue—everything but the eyeballs. Front and rear view of an Easter Island woman.

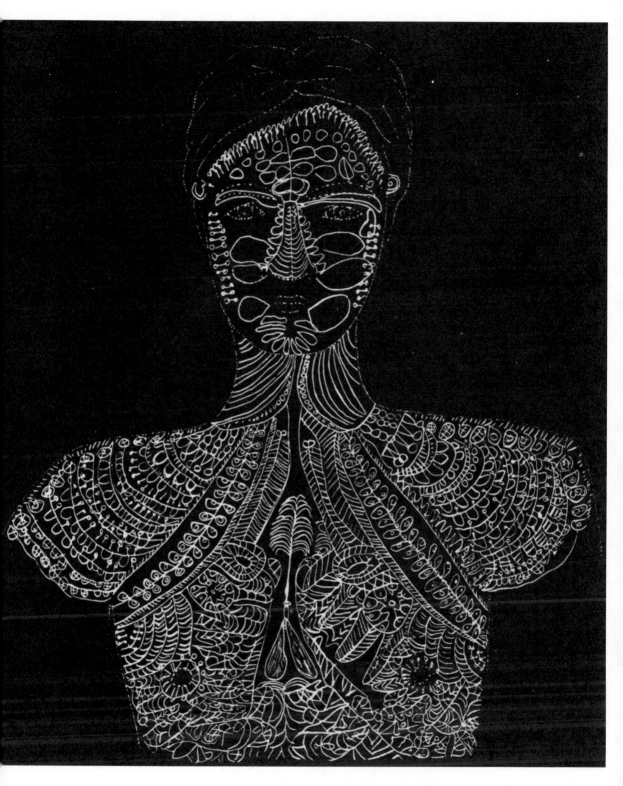

Sketch for a tattoo design made by a native of Easter Island.
From Abhandlungen und Berichte des Königlichen Zoologischen und
Anthropologisch-Ethnographischen Museums zu Dresden. *1899.*

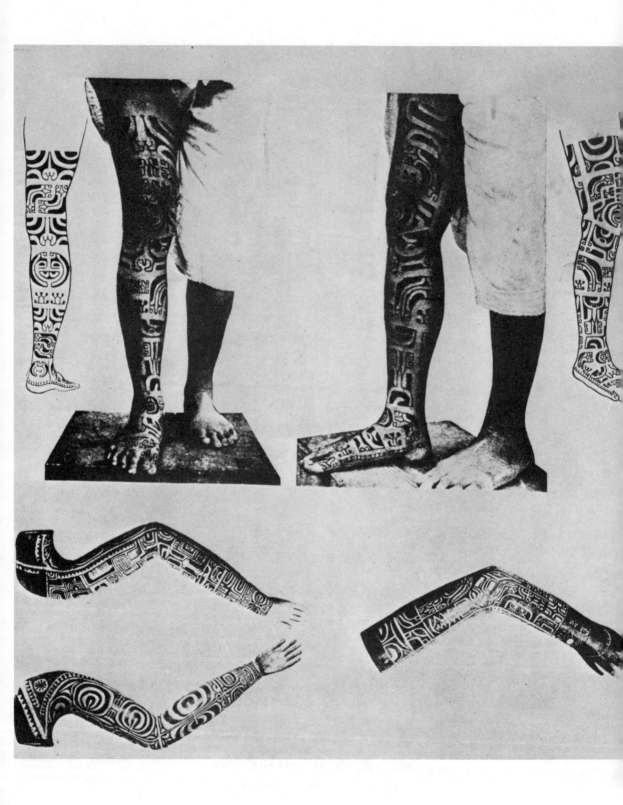

Marquesan tattoos from Die Marquesaner und ihre Kunst *by Karl von den Steinen.*

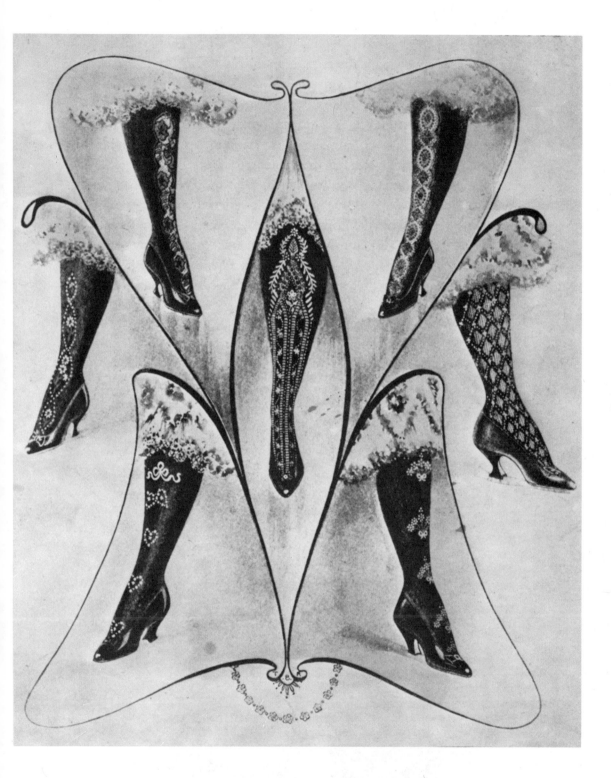

Industrial man shuns permanent decoration since it would interfere with the ever-repeating cycles of dress fashions. American stockings, 1902.

of primitive painting and tattooing suggest clothing. The larger the surface of decorated skin, the more it resembles a garment; it makes a person look more completely dressed than in scanty clothes. Tattooing especially achieves a sort of trompe-l'oeil effect in which the human skin is miraculously transformed into dry goods.

During its long history, tattooing was practiced by such dissimilar peoples as the Jews of old and the ancient Britons. "Not one great country," noted Darwin, "can be named, from the Polar regions in the north to New Zealand in the south, in which the aborigines do not tattoo themselves."[62] Perhaps because among us tattoo is not intended for public display, constituting an underground art, so to speak, it never developed beyond a limited repertory of symbolic and erotic stereotypes that are only a few rungs above gutter art.

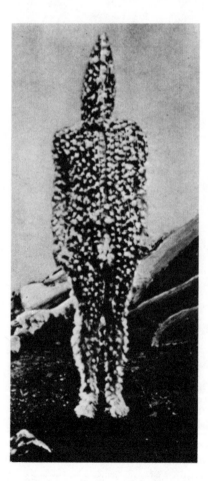 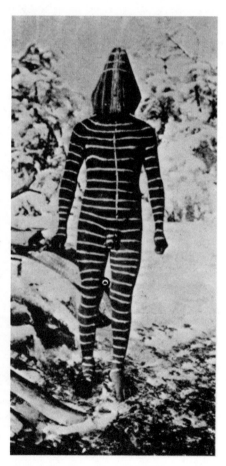

Fuegians from Feuerland Indianer *by Martin Gusinde.*

Paradoxically, tattoo's greatest drawback is its durability. Permanent, indeed indelible, unless a cumbersome process of erasure is brought into play, it does not fit in with the engineered obsolescence of the fashionable scene.

Generally speaking, body art has fallen on bad days; our mental climate is, and mostly has been, unfavorable to improvisation. Today's women never learned to weave wreaths of flowers for their lovers, as was the custom in those distant times that we ignorantly call the Dark Ages. Neither has an American male ever been known to festoon his sweetheart. These rites of spring, and the equally charming custom of forming sprigs and sprays into a kind of thatch for the head, are uncongenial to modern man. Yet it has not always been that way. In southern countries, where people are on easy terms with nature, floral decorations for man and beast have a long tradition. Traveling in Italy (in 1825) the British essayist William Hazlitt observed that "the people of both sexes in this country stick flowers in their hair, often with great taste." Dining in a small town near Venice, he noted with surprise that the waiter had ornamented his hair with ripe cherries, "a style of decoration more suitable for the ringlets of pretty girls." Flower or fruit trimmings on a male skull strike us as atavistic, not to say absurd; the picture of the tired businessman, his bald pate garnished with laurel, a bunch of grapes dangling over one ear, is quite beyond our imagination. A distinct mythological flavor with a strong suggestion of sin seems to cling to all live botanical specimens when summoned to decorate a man's body. Not that we deny him a *single* flower. However, etiquette relegates it to the buttonhole, the most wretched flower vase ever invented.

Only in those remote outposts of the nation, the Hawaiian Islands, does one come across flower-bedecked people. In fact, there they are a common sight. On close contact, however, they turn out to be professional entertainers working for the local Chamber of Commerce. Passengers debarking in the fiftieth state of the Union are draped by them, free of charge, with garlands of flowers, like prize-winning oxen at a country fair. These atavistic flower garlands are meant to please the eye as well as play on the sense of smell. And so they do—with a vengeance. The fragrance of tuberose—a prominent ingredient in Hawaiian leis—of gardenia, lily, and some other white flowers often produces voluptuous sensations in high-strung women. "Make the chastest woman smell the flowers she likes best," remarked Mantegazza, the author of the *Physiology of Love*, "and she will close her eyes, breathe deeply, and, if very sensitive, tremble all over, presenting an intimate picture which otherwise she never shows, except perhaps to her lover."

The dangers that lurk in fresh flowers can be avoided by trying to make do with artificial ones. They are used in profusion for garnishing women's hats, especially those worn in that tribal celebration, the Easter Parade. There, the flowery hat has become the secular symbol for a religious feast, much as Odin's sacred oak once made the transition to the Christmas tree. It mainly helps to turn fears into hopes; it serves as an elixir for the mind, a bulwark against the grim Easter weather and life in general.

At times—as in the nineteen-twenties when the *cloche* enjoyed popularity—hats were extremely simple without damaging women's

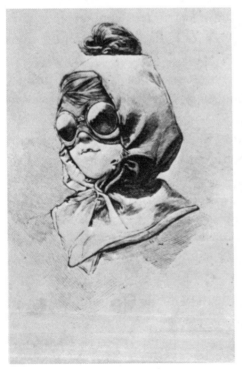
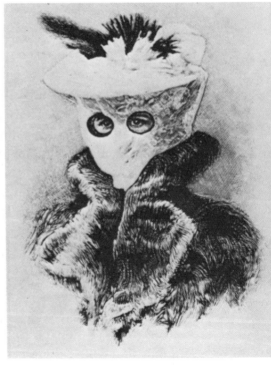

Two samples of French headgear for pioneering automobilists, 1903.

morale. Apparently, utilitarian principles do not enter into consideration; costume has to be evaluated against its historical background. The vogue for elephantine hats, for example, coincided with the advent of the motorcar, a vehicle that in its early days afforded practically no shelter from wind and rain, let alone from the dust of unpaved roads. A generation later, when automobiles had acquired the coziness of a boudoir, hats shrank to the plainness of potato peels.

In this country, men's hats lead a precarious existence since usages of salutation, or rather non-salutation, dispense with them as ceremonial objects. For whereas an old-world gentleman bares his head in greeting, Americans consider raising their hat to a person a deplorable holdover from feudal times. What did survive from the storehouse of costume history are hard hats. I do not mean bowlers or top hats but helmets—the colorful head coverings of our modern knights and highwaymen, the motorcyclists, construction and demolition workers. The noblest headgear of all, crowns and nimbuses, handsome and suggestive as they are,. have fallen into disuse in a world where true princes and saints are scarce.

Man's need for embellishment has drawn him toward ornaments less ephemeral than wreaths and garlands. The most obvious among decorative objects that call attention to himself are eyeglasses. Originally a crutch for the eye, glasses have made themselves accessory to mystification. It so happens that not only dark glasses help to blur a person's identity, transparent ones can be equally deceitful. "The awkward way that they catch the light and make the wearer look eyeless," wrote the author of an 1885 book on dress, "is known to all those who are fortunate enough to be exempt from these disagreeable adjuncts. It is difficult to understand, however, why people who are obliged by actual defective vision to resort to them should unnecessarily disfigure themselves by wearing rectangular or large round glasses, the eye, which they surround, being elliptical in form."[63] As we have noted earlier, some people wear glasses for the love of framing their eyes, regardless of the state of their eyesight. On the other hand, a person with only one eye impaired, who refuses to bespectacle the other, good one, in the United States experiences the wrath of popular prejudice that sees in the monocle the modern equivalent of the evil eye.

An even older aid in the game of hide-and-seek is the fan, now largely confined to oblivion. (The fan's definition as "an instrument held in the hand and used for raising a current of air to cool the face" is about as inclusive as calling the nose a peg from which to hang one's spectacles.) In everyday life its sight is as rare as that of an Indian's headdress, and although it is occasionally encountered in the ballroom as a badge of gentility, modern woman lacks the knack of putting it to good use. As a weapon in the heartless play by which she gained power over a man, it is to all intents and purposes passé. Like so many other relics of a once unhurried pace of life it has been laid to rest in the nation's attic, our museums.

During the five thousand years of its existence the fan has filled many needs, ceremonial and practical. It was indispensable for civic and religious rites, and in some countries it still is. One also has to keep in mind that it was never exclusively a woman's prerogative; men always had equal claims to it. In Japan, for instance, a country which nobody would call backward, the fan is still as popular as ever. Both sexes are in the habit of fanning themselves and each other. Although air conditioner and electric fan are common enough, they have not displaced the traditional, hand-manipulated paper fan. The breeze it generates may be trifling compared to ventilation by mechanical means yet the satisfaction derived from its extensional quality by far outweighs its utilitarian function. Besides, the fan-empowered hand speaks a silent but pithy language. In times past, the condemned criminal walking to his execution demonstrated non-chalance by vigorously fanning himself. Similarly, the Japanese bridegroom I observed toying with his fan during the wedding cere-mony in a New York church expressed in pantomime the legendary stoicism of his race.

Another plaything for idle hands is the pipe. A semi-functional part-time head ornament with a simple but nevertheless unpredict-able mechanism, it has gained much favor in recent years. Originally a container for burning tobacco, today it is chiefly used as a tran-quilizer that induces slow gesturing and a more accentuated though less intelligible speech. Men attach as much importance to its shape and color as women do to the right shade of lipstick. Not only does the pipe complement a man's facial features, it greatly bolsters his ego. A pipe in the secure grip of his teeth symbolizes meditative reflection, mature deliberation and superiority in general.

Lastly, when it comes to camouflaging one's self; to literally changing one's true colors, the most marked effect is achieved by dyeing one's hair. Apart from granting a reprieve from aging, every new hair color raises hopes for a better self. Racial as well as sexual traits have been ascribed to various shades of hair and although no two opinions agree on the subject, popular sentiment has always linked certain hair colors to sex appeal. So do operatic libretti with their archetypes of human character; dark hair is standard equipment for *femmes fatales*. Salome, Kundry, Carmen, the temptresses in the grand manner, are all brunettes. Tepid and frigid women, although perhaps no less toxic, are usually represented as blondes. Whatever the reasons for our bias in favor of fair hair, the larger part of the world does not agree with us. A good many races are partial to dark hair. To the Japanese, for instance, a fair-skinned nation, only black hair looks beautiful; when they encountered Europeans for the first time, they dubbed them "red devils" because of their light hair, and even today a blond foreigner evokes sentiments of pity.

They are not the only ones to whom the possession of light hair seems a misfortune. Bishop James of Nisibis, a holy man who lived in the fourth century A.D., is remembered by a miraculous, albeit spiteful, act of hair-dyeing. Once while passing a fountain where young women were washing their linen, he was shocked by the décolletage they permitted themselves at work. Convinced that this assault on his modesty called for retaliation, he cursed the women and, for good measure, the fountain as well. The latter dried up instantly, while the women's hair changed from black to a "sandy" color.

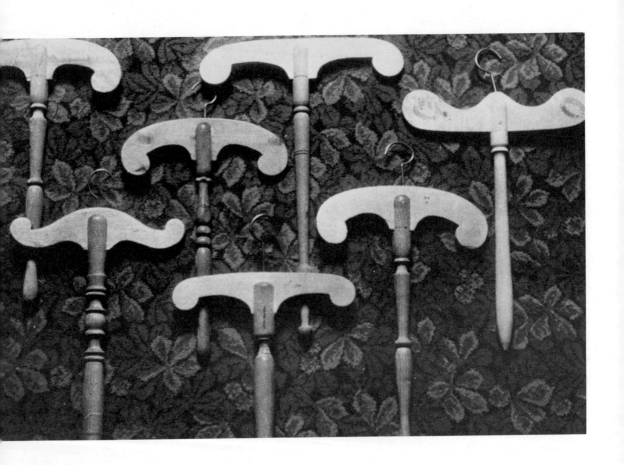

*The shapes of clothes hangers at a first-class hotel in Florence might prompt
future generations of anatomists to jump to highly erroneous conclusions about
a twentieth-century Tuscan's physique.*

Cut and dry goods

When making a jacket, the tailor—a trompe-l'oeil artist without
fear and reproach—or for that matter, the garment manufacturer,
more than compensate for what nature withheld. Even a physique
about as articulate as a bag of potatoes in their hands becomes endowed with shoulders and a waist. The shape is the thing and by no
means the human shape. However pliant the material, some measure
of doubling, lining and padding helps to mold it into a shell that for
a while stands for the image of perfection—a glorified abstraction of
man's better self. Since our concept of the human anatomy is subject
to endless revisions, the silhouette may change from year to year.
What does not change is our idea of the tailored suit as a hollow
casting of man.

This school of thought and its consistent application to apparel
has its disadvantages. Once off the back of their owner, clothes ought
to be kept on dummies to preserve their shape. Instead they are put
on hangers which, as we know, are no substitute for even the most
wretched pair of shoulders. Some will spoil the "best-fitting" suit,
an occurrence by no means rare. The calamity is multiplied and
magnified in those purgatories for clothes, the checkrooms of theaters
and restaurants, where insult is added to injury by exacting payment

for damages inflicted. Not that clothes fare any better in the home. A foreigner unversed in our folkways is dismayed to see his hat and overcoat as roughly treated at a friend's house as in a public place. According to custom, the guests' clothes, some perhaps still wet from snow or rain, are carried to the bedroom and piled unceremoniously upon the matrimonial bed. On leaving, the guest may find himself trying to extricate his belongings from a heap of promiscuous garments, much like scavenging in a garbage dump. Happily, such abuse has its positive side. Vandalism, like waste, far from being condemned, has always been regarded as a prime mover of our economy. Traditional mistreatment—particularly by children—of our most intimate shelter, clothes, reflects our general attitude towards the environment at large.

Clothes more tractable than ours are of course nothing new. Clothes that represent a perfect unity of form and substance once were common in most civilized countries, and still are worn in parts of Asia, Africa and America. In a way, sari, sarong, and rebozo—to mention only some of the better known geometric types—are the equivalent of dress in classical antiquity. Since the latter has been exhaustively treated in quite a number of books, it will serve our purpose to sum up its chief merits:

Instead of starting out with yardgoods as we do, the ancients made their clothes from uncut lengths of material. The exact amount that went into a garment was loomed at home, much as a self-respecting Italian housewife makes her own pasta. At any rate, such was the procedure in earliest times. There was no wastage, there were no scraps. Cloth *was* clothing (whereas our method of making a dress calls for cutting a dress fabric into pieces, only to join these pieces together according to the cabalistic rules of dressmaking). It fell of its own weight from the shoulders. Never intended to "fit" the human form, it had no need for seams, hems, and darts. Devoid of buttons and buttonholes, the stigmata of modern dress, it was held in place with a fibula or two, the prototype of our safety pin. Or it might be tied at the shoulders, under the breasts or, to produce an overfold, around the waist. But the point is that it escaped dressmaking's pitfalls.

The effect of so much artlessness was anything but poor. The

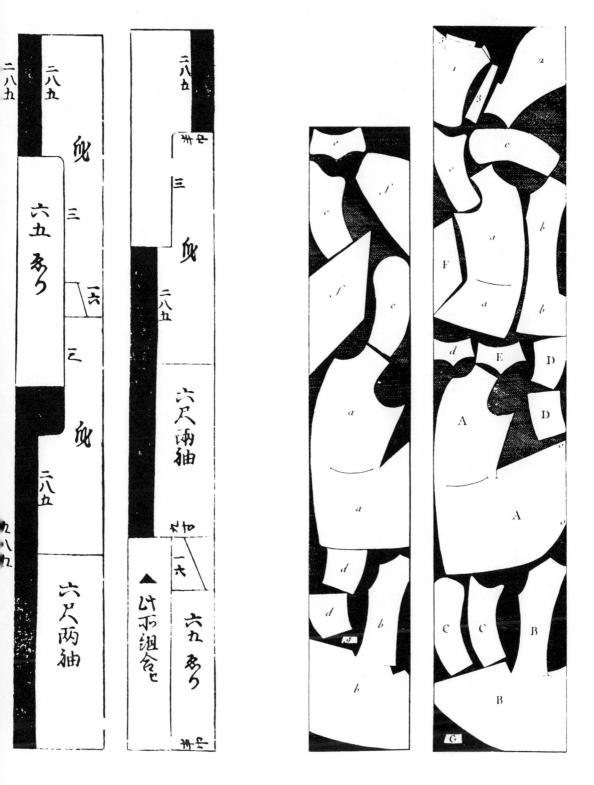

Two pattern books, published only five years apart, illustrate the proverbial incompatibility of East and West. The Japanese manual, How To Cut Silk, 1764, teaches a rational approach to dress construction which results in utmost economy, whereas the wasteful ways of the Art du Tailleur, 1769, call for reducing a fabric to scrap.

loosely wrapped garments were never as regimented as most costume books would like us to believe, for even though classical costume can be reduced to a few basic shapes, the manner in which it was worn resulted in a great variety of what in the garment trade is known as "styles." The best-dressed woman was she who knew best how to wear her garment, who had grace and charm, qualities unrelated to social and economic status. In other words, dress was a tangible expression of democracy, a concept that defies translation into our world of thought.

Although during the past thousand years no climatic changes occurred in Europe that would have warranted radically different clothes, the geometric types of costume disappeared with the civilizations that produced them. What did change was the outlook on life.

When the antique world began to totter with agonizing slowness to its fall; when barbaric tribes from the North and East began to press upon it from without, and spreading Christianity rebelled from within, the centuries-old traditions fell into neglect. Gods and demigods of old were transmogrified into legions of saints, and men came to regard life on earth as a way station on the road to hell (or heaven). With people forever famished for drama, connoisseurship of human beauty, male and female, shifted to a clinical curiosity about human endurance tests undergone by torture, a subject that was to become of paramount interest, not to say an obsession, in religious art. A crucified man displaced the thousand and one Olympian images of the acceptance of life. Holy pictures expounded on the best methods on how to burn, quarter, break on the wheel, or otherwise mangle a human being, and on the equally complicated torments of the damned in purgatory. In short, torture emerged as one among the more entertaining aspects of the new faith. The nude that had been exorcised to a certain extent from the public bath by ecclesiastic and mundane authorities alike, crept back into circulation under the guise of the martyr and the hermit. In the penumbra of a chapel, Saint Sebastian triumphed on canvas and in stone as a glorified pinup of the pious, while Adam and Eve, the perennial exhibitionists, could always be depended upon to rescue nakedness from oblivion. In plain daylight, however, the human body was carefully hidden from sight. Clothes were hermetic.

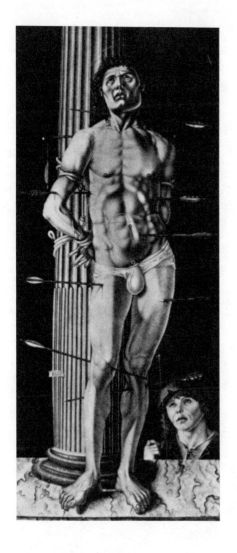

The sensuousness that pervades certain images of saints often equals that of ancient pagan idols. Gleaming like a baroque pearl, the package of San Sebastian's genitals cannot but mesmerize the pious. The painting by Antonio Mainieri now hangs in the Pinacoteca Nazionale in Bologna.

The barbarian invaders brought an entirely new concept of dress into this self-contained world. Hunters and nomads that they were, they borrowed their clothes from the animals by literally peeling the skin off their backs. The resulting garments, pieced together from pelts and hides, had their good points; they shed water and provided warmth and camouflage. Like a second skin they followed the human form. In time they grew their ugly excrescences, our arm- and leg-sleeves, and I for one am inclined to believe that they were suggested by a hide's natural extensions that covered an animal's four legs. The joining of odd-shaped pieces resulted in con-

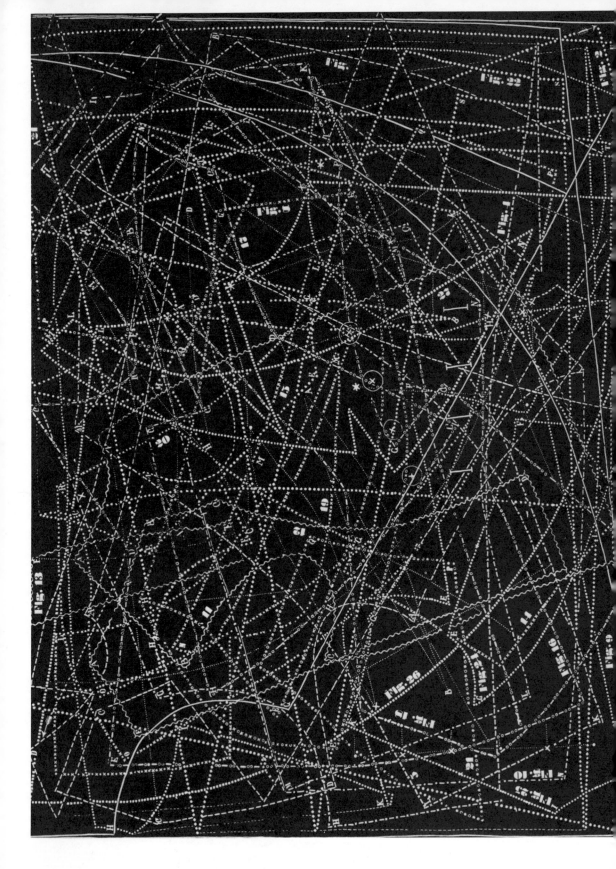

The page from an 1873 pattern book for housewives and seamstresses is a document
of considerable interest. Apart from affording some insight into our sartorial
conceits, it is a silent comment on industrial man's state of mind.

siderable waste, and the need to economize led to pattern making. This custom was by no means abandoned when, subsequently, clothes were made from textiles. Indeed, it persists to our day. Whether we like it or not, our jackets and trousers are inventions of the bronze age.

Neither was the cut of trousers improved by the transition from hides to yardgoods. Trousers represent a typical paradox of modern dress—an abstract shape, the tube, superimposed upon an organic shape, the leg. The trinity of thigh, knee and calf, each marvelously molded and replete with eye and sex appeal, is stuck into a cylinder that would be just right for a peg leg but fails to do justice to a live one. As packaging jobs go, the result is ludicrous and not a little sad. "The great tragedy of the average man's life," said Bernard Shaw, "is that Nature refuses to conform to the cylindrical ideal, and when the marks of his knees and elbows begin to appear he is filled with shame."[64]

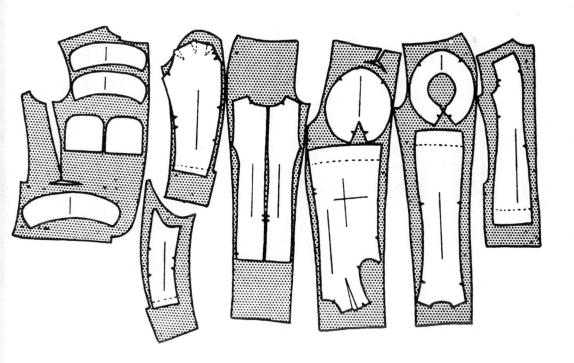

Modern man's mentality is graphically expressed in these instructions for making a child's outfit from the ruins of father's suit. What looks like a sample of the art of the insane, is indeed a page from a government publication, Leaflet No. 230, U.S. Department of Agriculture.

The trouser crease, introduced about the turn of the century and intended to remedy this calamity, made things worse. Its sole function seems to consist of reminding us that trouser legs are not for bending; to the tailor's mind the perfect gentleman is a stiff-legged man. The pioneer-architect Adolf Loos—a man with two average legs but more than average contempt for the day's fashions—had his own ideas about dress and never hesitated to put them to the test. As far as trousers were concerned, he wore them creased sidelong. The crease, instead of occupying its customary prowlike position, followed the seam of the trouser leg.

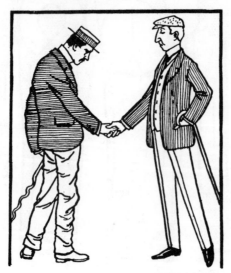
The introduction of the trouser crease brought no lasting improvement to the modish silhouette since goose stepping—which is the only way to walk without disturbing the crease—was never made compulsory. Advertisement.

158

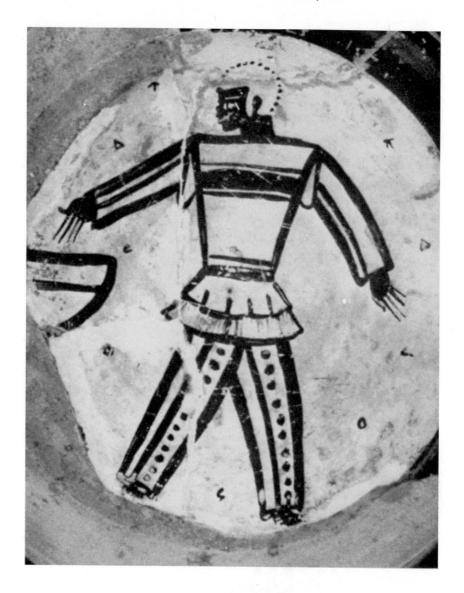

The shape of present-day men's clothes goes back to the beginning of the French revolution, when a social taboo was attached to knee breeches and stockings, and ankle-length trousers were promoted to a proletarian attribute. Whatever the reasons that made Frenchmen select trousers as the visible proof of their newly gained freedom, it strikes one as ironic that they should have modeled them after the costume of Italian buffoons. Through all the vagaries of dress, the tubular pants of the Barbarians survived on the stage as the hallmark of comic actors. In fact, the word "pants"—short for pantaloons—honors the memory of Pantalone, the top clown of the Commedia dell' Arte. John Evelyn, in his *Tyrannus or the Mode,* a "gentle satyr" (as he called it), published in 1661, called pantaloons "a kind of Hermaphrodite and of neither Sex."[65] (I shall get back to their bisexual nature in a minute.) Whatever the more profound theories about the origin of trousers, Pantalone, Brighella, and Arlequino—before the latter adopted the patchwork harlequin costume that carries his name—anticipated the modern business suit by several centuries.

Three generations ago, tubular dress was by no means as unanimously accepted as it is today, and protests against its inconvenience

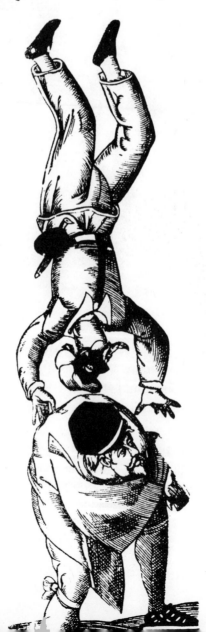

The name of Pantalone, a character of the commedia dell'arte, survives in our word pants.

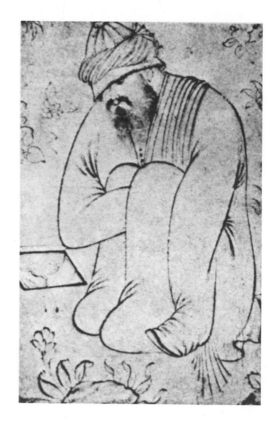

Dervish. Sixteenth century.
From Frederick Robert Martin,
The miniature paintings and
painters of Persia.

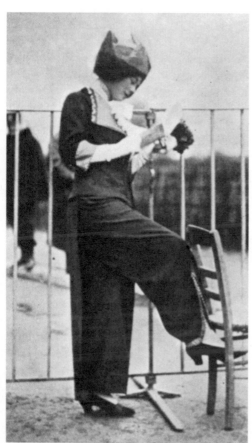

French trouser skirt, c. 1912.
From Alfred Holtmont,
Die Hosenrolle.

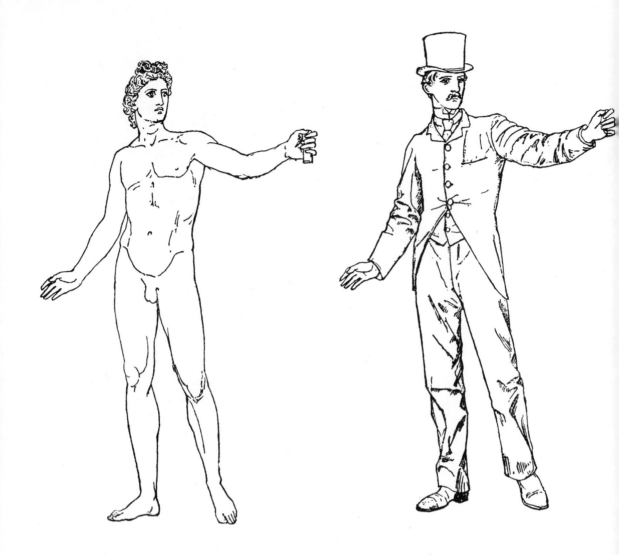

and ugliness were the order of the day. "Whether tailoring," wrote one malcontent in an English periodical in 1893, "suggested the merits of the tube to engineers as affording the highest degree of rigidity with a given amount of material, or whether engineering suggested it to tailors, must be left to the investigation of the careful historian." (The last word has not been said about the woolly tube; its principle, however, has been generally recognized and is being applied to dress with a perseverance worthy of a better cause.) "The tube," our correspondent went on, "is not full enough to take any folds of its own, but it is just full enough to miss all the lines of the figure. And this dismal, tasteless, graceless type of form has allied itself to an equally dismal, tasteless, lifeless type of color. We have become so inured to this state of things that we regard it as normal, and fancy any infusion of grace or color into our dress would be phantastic and unbusinesslike, forgetting that there have been good men of business in Venice, Florence, in the Netherlands, etc., who did not find dingy suits or battered tubes essential to success in their mercantile pursuits; forgetting that never till this century was so degraded a type of dress worn anywhere, and now only in 'civilized' Europe, America, and the colonies."[66] To judge from this outburst, men of three generations ago were not only more articulate in their pronouncements on dress than we are today, they actually smarted under its ignominy. Yet not in their gloomiest mood could they have anticipated a century-long dominance of undertakers' clothes.

The continuing success of tubular male dress, so devoid of appeal, particularly sex appeal—if we prefer to disregard the meanings projected into it by psychoanalysis—is paralleled only by that of the skirt. Skirts came into use long before people wore any other articles of dress. The earliest fashion plates, prehistoric paintings, show women dressed in long skirts, bare from the waist up. The skirt's lasting popularity is understandable: it helps to counterbalance the notorious topheaviness of the human figure, a defect that has plagued artists of all times. Anybody with an eye for proportion

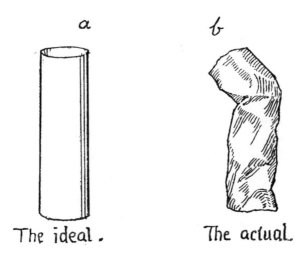

a   *b*

The ideal.   The actual.

Opposite and above, four drawings from an article on tubular dress in the English Illustrated Magazine, *1893.*

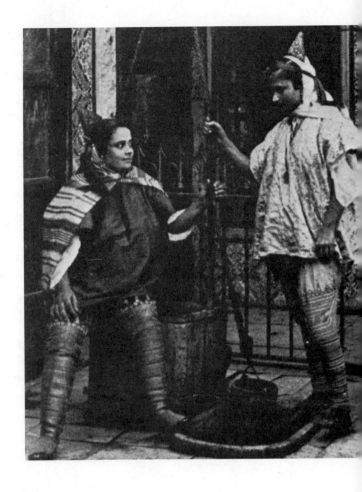

can see that our bodies' center of gravity is misplaced. An elementary expedient for correcting this shortcoming consists, as we shall see later, of putting a woman on pedestals, thus adding inches to her height. Another requires raising her waistline to under her breasts. The third universal remedy calls for wrapping her legs in a long skirt. Apart from optically improving her figure, this produces a pleasing sculptural effect. As Flügel put it, "instead of being supported on just two legs with nothing but thin air between them, a skirted human being assumes much more ample and voluminous proportions, and the space between the legs is filled up, often with great increase of dignity."[67] (The theory that attributes the cause for hiding the legs to modesty does not explain the prevalence of ankle-length skirts in cave paintings. Whatever may have been the

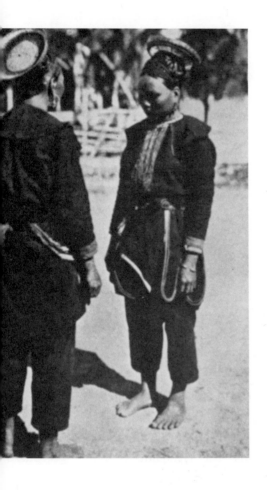
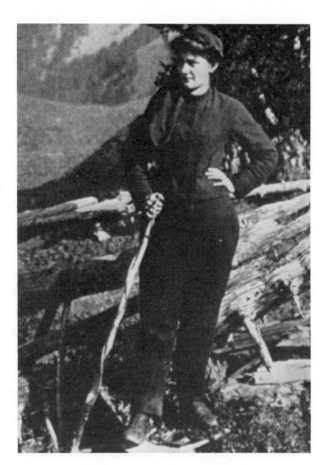

symptoms of good breeding in those remote times, it seems that a short skirt should have met the demands of prehistoric etiquette.)

Sex has been so obviously the mainspring of clothes invention that one cannot help being puzzled by the purported asexual character of the skirt. No doubt, in this respect the skirt represents an anomaly among garments. Any inquiry into the nature of modern clothes therefore must take into account our arbitrary separation of garments into male and female ones. For what to us may seem to be a matter of course, to others is a mere whim. The idea that the anatomical differences between man and woman justify the need for different garments is not substantiated by history. In the past, there often was little or no distinction between male and female dress. With a few exceptions, the early Greeks had no special clothes for the sexes, nor had the Persians and early Assyrians. The Hebrews, too, were content with identical garments for men and women and, on the authority of Tacitus, so were the Teutons. And why not? Neck, shoulders, and waist, the three main points of attachment for dress, are alike in man and woman. Sexual characteristics, once they are covered, would seem to make dual dress unnecessary. Even today, some people who perform heavy labor are not affected by these problems; in the Austrian and Swiss Alps for instance, many peasant women wear trousers in preference to skirts, and have been doing so for ages. Trousers for women are also essential in workshops where machines endanger a worker clad in skirts. Moreover, in the Orient, female trousers are practically the rule. From one end of Asia to the other, from Turkish pantaloons to Japanese *mompe*, women have worn and are still wearing bifurcated garments, at least in the strongholds of native culture.

And what are we to make of civilizations that either show a complete reversal of our dress habits, or where people are unconcerned with the question of what sort of dress is appropriate for man, what sort for woman? Do we accuse an Arab of being effeminate because he wears ladylike garments, a flapping headcloth, and barefoot sandals? We certainly do not. The notion that a man's legs ought to be enclosed separately belongs to an age that was reluctant to acknowledge the existence of women's legs, when the word leg was taboo in polite society, and women limped through life on limbs. Indeed, the idea that bifurcated garments belong to man and skirts to women is purely arbitrary. Throughout the history of mankind, probably more men wore skirts, more women wore trousers. If anything, man's most precious ornament is better hidden in the folds of a skirt. Or so it seemed until the analyst gave dress one hard look. After that, nothing was quite the same any more.

Volumes of learned dissertations have been written on the alleged significance of anything from a buttonhole to a Van Dyke beard, and to believe the authors, dress is a hotbed of sexuality. Anybody even slightly acquainted with their articles of faith can identify trousers, sleeves, collars, and hats as phallic symbols. To top it all, the shoe is professed to be not just a phallic or a uterine symbol; it is both. To grasp its full meaning; to fathom the power

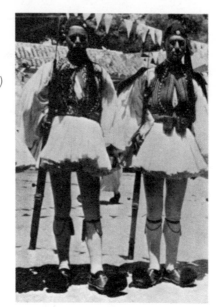

Evzones. (Courtesy, Greek Office of Information)

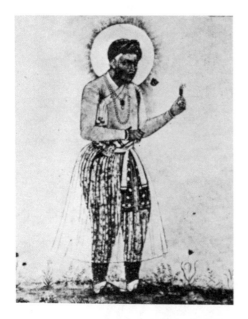

Indian courtier. Seventeenth century.
From Frederick Robert Martin,
The miniature paintings and painters of Persia.

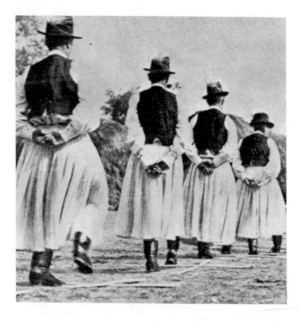

Hungarian peasants.
From Béla Paulini, The Pearly Bouquet.

it exerts on the human mind, the shoe has to be broken down into its components—the stiff and soft, the convex and concave parts—which in turn have to be scrutinized for *their* special meaning.

Sexual implications multiply when dress meets body. To give just one example—according to our sartorial tradition, the overlap of a garment determines its sex. By buttoning it to the right it becomes suitable for men only. Women button to the left. There is no explication for this custom except that in European folklore the right side of the body has always been considered male, the left side female. "Right" is the proper and just side; "left" the wrong side; *gauche* means both left and uncouth. The rest of the world does not share this belief; in the Far East, where the overlap made its appearance much earlier than in the West, the kimono, for instance, always overlaps to the right, regardless of whether it is worn by man or woman. In its homeland, the kimono is a male garment, and no lapping to the left will make it female. Only the kimono of the dead overlaps to the left.

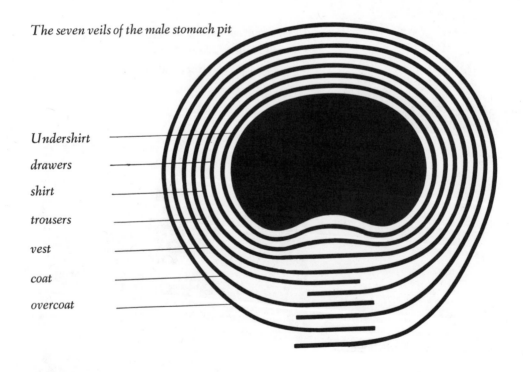

The seven veils of the male stomach pit

Undershirt

drawers

shirt

trousers

vest

coat

overcoat

Sometimes these whimsical rules are upset by innovations. Slide fastener and snap button, the only dress fastenings invented in the past eight hundred years, have muddled the picture. Eliminating as it does the overlap, the slidefastener gives no cue to a garment's sex. However, the question whether a dress, or part of a dress, is male, female, or neutral, is not for the individual to decide. While a man is free to indulge in cross-dressing at home, in public he is not. Although our society has relaxed, if not altogether rescinded, its prejudice against trousered women, a man wearing a skirt in the street invites arrest. If he must, he had better choose a folk costume; anything from an Evzone's miniskirt to an Oriental's trailing robe will make him acceptable to the ultimate arbiter, the policeman.

In the distant past, the interchange of clothes between the sexes was not thought to be unnatural or sinful. Rather it was looked upon as part of amatory play or popular amusement. During the Roman Saturnalia, the three December holidays in honor of the god Saturnius, when the humdrum daily routine was temporarily set aside and master and slave exchanged rôles, men dressed as women, and vice versa. Throughout the Middle Ages, cross-dressing was one of carnival's pleasures, and still later, it was carried over to the stage. In baroque opera, which was largely written for female voices, the protagonists are irresistibly driven either to adopt each other's clothes, or to fall in love with disguised partners. Elizabethan drama thrives on transvestism. In a play by Lyly for example, two women disguised as men fall in love with each other, each believing the other to be a man. (A happy end is engineered by dea ex machina Venus who changes one of the women into a man.) Another play has a man impersonating a woman who plays a man disguised as a woman. Surely, we are too obtuse to follow such involved plots, too lazy to bother about sexual metamorphosis through dress. Least of all do we understand the raptures of lovers caused by the exchange of their garments. The custom goes back to antiquity and was, or still is, alive on some Asian islands, the last holdouts against westernization, where the bridegroom puts on the garments which the bride has taken off. In our matriarchy, where women usurp men's clothes with impunity—and without thrilling to any erotic impact—men with a craving for female attire have to content themselves with the old-fashioned house gown, that most neutral piece of contemporary apparel. Withal, female clothes are becoming progressively desexed, if not altogether masculinized. For what else was the miniskirt of the late nineteen-sixties but the revived doublet of the fifteenth century?

In concept and character, many contemporary men's clothes belong to an era of gaslight and horse-drawn carriages—museum pieces that only an aficionado of costume can fully appreciate. Cuffs, collars, lapels, tabs, tails, and an incurable rash of buttons whose original functions have been forgotten and whose usefulness has been exhausted, are stubbornly preserved in a more or less atrophied state. Like the vastly unnecessary lapels, the jacket's collar is but a decorative rudiment. Its underside reveals a piece of incongruous material, which implies that the collar is not supposed to be turned up. Neither are the ends of a sleeve meant to be turned back, although several buttons (sometimes with corresponding buttonholes) are much in evidence. Yet the slits are missing from ready-made clothes. In sum, while buttons started out as fastenings, they ended up as the cheapest of ornaments.

To us, buttons are what glass beads were to the savage before he took an interest in traveler's checks. Although they have disappeared from shoes and from the fly of pants, there are times when they break out all over our clothes. Even in lean years, they hold their own; the inventory of a complete male outfit—shirt, trousers, vest, coat, and overcoat—yields dozens of buttons, functional, magical, and otherwise. The extra buttons of a double-breasted suit are as useless as a man's nipples, which probably inspired them in the first place. Few ever come to rest in a buttonhole; some remain forever at large, which makes them twice as vulnerable. Thanks to mechanized cleaning methods, they break or come loose; buttonholes are apt to contract a disease similar to scurvy.

Equally popular are pockets of every description. The fully dressed man has at his disposal about one and a half dozen pockets. Assuming that he were a conscientious man—a true believer in pockets as useful appendages—and wanted to fill them all, he would be hard put to find enough cargo. Moreover, since the ballast

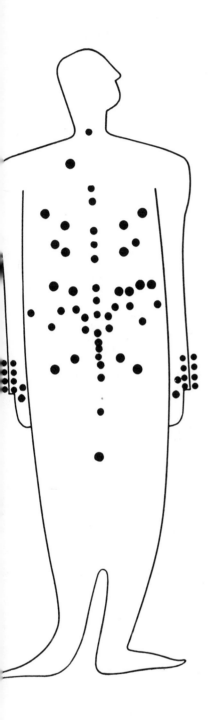
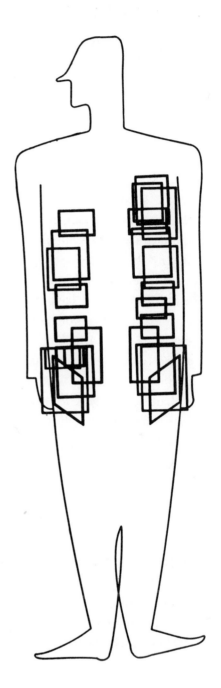

Only thirty years ago a fully clothed man's outfit was equipped with
seventy or more buttons and about two dozen pockets, most of them useless.

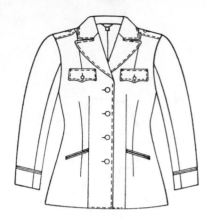

Four fake pockets on a modern uniform.
From Quartermaster Corps Specifications.

would seriously injure his sartorial silhouette, fashion decrees that the well-dressed man make little or no use of his pockets. Some of them are purely symbolic, to be conveniently ignored. Others are downright illusory. Such were the make-believe pockets of World War II female uniforms. Wacs and Waves sported two fake pockets with button-down flaps over the breasts, and two tightly sewn slits at waist height, all of them intractably virginal. How did the ladies manage? The passage of time has dimmed my memory to the point where it is difficult to recall whether they were allowed to carry handbags.

During the past hundred years, the soldier's uniform, once the apex of sartorial seductiveness, has been steadily declining in eye appeal. Darwin's dictum that "beauty is sometimes more important than success in battle," still held true in 1871, yet that very year marked the beginning of the end of the beautifully dressed combatant. At the outbreak of the Franco-Prussian war, the French hastened to abolish the infantryman's traditional red trousers, a target as perfect as the red jacket of the hunter. And long before horses gave way to tanks, the cavalry's gorgeous attire went on the scrap heap.

Of course, the conspicuous color of military clothes was never thought to be altogether unfunctional. It inspired pride in the good soldier; it was meant to make him aggressive. Just as male birds of a luxuriant plumage are more quarrelsome than dull-colored ones, the grandly attired elite troups always outdid ordinary soldiers in bravery. However, with methods of killing becoming increasingly impersonal, color was drained from uniforms until they resembled mechanics' outfits. If anything, modern uniforms have taken on the protective coloring of no man's land, blending the soldier into the warscape. The shadow dress of camouflage is worn to *escape* the enemy's notice; to approach him unobserved. A savage cosmetic touch, blackface, transforms the soldier—or so he hopes—into a specter. The ultimate metamorphosis will be accomplished by a piece of apparel to be reinvented—the tarn cap of legend, the magical hood of invisibility.

Footwear, the civilian's curse, sometimes becomes the soldier's doom. In the early stages of the 1941 Malayan campaign, British soldiers, deprived of motor transportation and unable to flee because their boots had crippled them, died by the thousands in prison camps. No foot troubles plagued the Japanese who always could steal a march on the enemy. Their uncanny way of sneaking up on their victims like jungle cats was attributed by our baffled soldiers to a new secret weapon—soft-soled digital socks that made for a noiseless, catlike walk. These socks had not, as was then believed, been expressly designed for modern warfare but were the farmer's traditional footgear for work in the rice paddies.

To be sure, all kinds of apparel for special duty have been devised over the years to meet new demands. It is doubtful though whether such novelties will find application for the civilian's wardrobe. Even space travel clothes do not feature any radical innovations, except perhaps the built-in privy. However, what strikes one at first as progress, turns out to be a retrograde step. The first astronauts' pants marked a return to the clothes of infancy when soiling one's diapers was not only permissible but *comme il faut*.

Can we then expect, historical evidence to the contrary, that unprecedented forms of apparel or, better yet, entirely new types of clothes will be invented in the near future? Turning the pages of a costume book, a fashion magazine, one senses instinctively that the creation of dress is not our forte. Surely there must be more to it. If clothes are meant to increase our attractiveness, indeed, our seductiveness, designers as well as makers of apparel have been singularly timid.

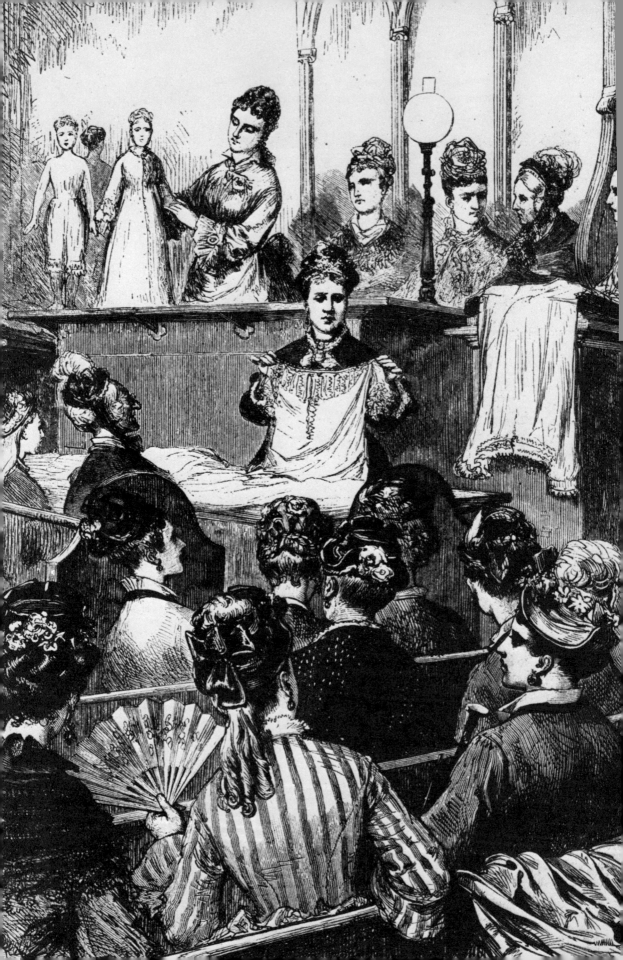

Dress reform and reform dress

The period that nostalgia dubbed the Gay Nineties, the heyday of American savoir-vivre and conspicuous display, was equally notorious for conspicuous filth. Even if bathing had appealed to the citizenry, it was hardly feasible for lack of tubs and the scarcity of water. New York hotels offered their guests just enough water for washing hands and face, and tenements had no provisions for bathing altogether; the stench of humanity was fearful. The streets, then as now littered with refuse and dog excrement, were swept less by the street cleaners' brooms than by women's skirts. "In 1900," says the *Britannica*, "one could not breathe freely for the dust raised by skirts." A contemporary witness has handed down to us the following snapshot: A lady, attired in a dress with a train that answered the fashion of the day, boarded a cab after a short walk, and left on the curbstone the rubbish she had collected while inadvertently sweeping the street. Our observer who had an analytical mind, made on the spot a quick inventory of the yield: Two cigar ends, nine cigarette ends, a portion of pork pie, four toothpicks, two hairpins, a stem of a clay pipe, three fragments of orange peel, one slice of cat's meat, half a sole of a boot, a plug of tobacco (chewed), straw, mud, scraps of paper, and miscellaneous street refuse.[68]

American dress reformers sought sanctuary in consecrated places, much as rebels
do today. This meeting was conducted in 1874 in Boston's Freeman Place Chapel.
Courtesy, Picture Collection, New York Public Library)

Sporadic attempts to improve the hygienic quality of dress go back to the eighteenth century, yet neither dressmakers nor physicians to whom the urge to do something about a more intelligent clothes construction would seem to come natural, had enough imagination or critical sense. Whereas a knowledge of food and food preparation always marked the true gentleman, any interest he showed in the dress of the opposite sex that went beyond its erotic attraction, brought suspicion or ridicule upon him. Thus the American dress-reform movement of the second half of the nineteenth century was started and fought to its inglorious end almost entirely by women whose energies were largely misdirected. Men regarded it as a comic incident or, at best, a concomitant of the temperance and woman suffrage movement.

Unfortunately, the women who had banded together to find ways of escaping the tyranny of trailing skirts stopped short of inventing radically new garments. As they themselves admitted, "We propose no particular costume"; in fact, none of them seem to have attempted to investigate the anatomy of dress. All they could think of was the universal and unconditional introduction of shorter skirts and trousers for women. It was no coincidence that they turned to the East, the acknowledged fountainhead of wisdom and pleasure, where the dress of the sexes is usually reversed, where women wear trousers as a badge of femininity. "In patrist periods," wrote Gordon Rattray Taylor (*Sex in History*), "men dress in a style quite different from that adopted by women; while in matrist periods it is sometimes difficult to tell them apart. It is as if the patrist was so determined not to be taken for a woman that he exaggerates all his masculine attributes and minimizes all his feminine ones. Furthermore, he forces his womenfolk into an exaggerated femininity, magnifying their relative weakness into complete helplessness."[69]

The papers that were read in the assemblies of the reformers, or published in the pages of progressive periodicals, compensated by their forcefulness of argumentation for what they lacked in insight. "Nature," maintained one dissident, "never intended that the sexes should be distinguished by apparel." (She did not bother to disclose her source of information.) "The beard," she went on, "which was assigned solely to man, is the natural token of sex. But man effeminates himself, contrary to the purpose of nature, by shaving off his beard; and then, lest his sex should be mistaken, he arrogates to himself a particular form of dress, the wearing of which by the female sex he declares to be grave misdemeanor."[70] This did not go over well with the guardians of the official morality who regarded wearing trousers as men's inalienable right. Clergymen, unwilling to miss the opportunity for throwing The Book at the mutinous women, quoted Deut. XXII, 5: "The woman shall not wear what pertaineth unto a man." Of course, had American women been better acquainted with Bible history, they would have been able to

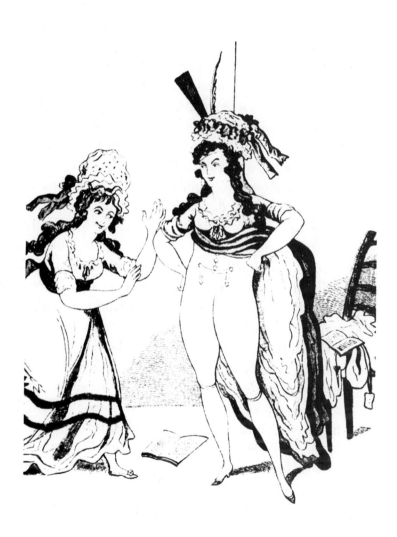

"Her brother's trousers,"
drawing by Richard Newton.

retort that in Moses' time it was precisely the women who wore the pants. None of them questioned the priests' right to wear skirts.

One panelist pointed out, quite correctly, that "dress is the most complex and difficult of all arts; for resting on the framework of the human body, an adjunct and accomplice in all man's expression, it requires the broadest knowledge of humanity and of individuality to understand its mysteries."[71] Alas, such knowledge was in short supply. As a rule, the reformers did not go beyond lamenting their misfortune and pilloring the absurdity of current dress styles: "When I see a woman climbing upstairs with her baby in one arm, and its bowl of bread and milk in the other, and see her tripping on her dress at every stair (if, indeed, baby, bowl, bread, milk, and mother do not go down in universal chaos), it is only from the efforts of long skill and experience on the part of the mother in performing that acrobatic feat."[72]

The event that fused female discontent and brought trousers, or, as they were to be called, bloomers, into the world, was not, as might be expected today, a well-publicized fashion show but the casual encounter of several like-minded women in a country house in northern New York State. The introduction of bifurcated garments to American womanhood was described by Mrs. Bloomer herself, mainly to dispel the belief that she had invented the costume that was to bear her name. "In March, 1851," she wrote, "Elizabeth Smith Miller, daughter of Hon. Gerrit Smith of Peterboro, N.Y., visited her cousin, Elizabeth Cady Stanton, at Seneca Falls, N.Y., which was then my home and where I was publishing the *Lily*, America's mouth-piece of feminism, and where Mrs. Stanton also resided. Mrs. Miller came to us in a short skirt and full Turkish trousers, a style of dress she had been wearing some two months. The matter of woman's dress having been just previously discussed in the *Lily*, Mrs. Miller's appearance led Mrs. Stanton to at once adopt a style, and I very soon followed, Mrs. Stanton introducing it to Seneca Falls' public two or three days in advance of me."[73] From the detailed accounts that appeared in the papers we can form a fairly accurate picture of the new garment, as well as of the public's reaction to it. Mrs. Bloomer's first costume consisted of a dress of red and black silk that reached a few inches

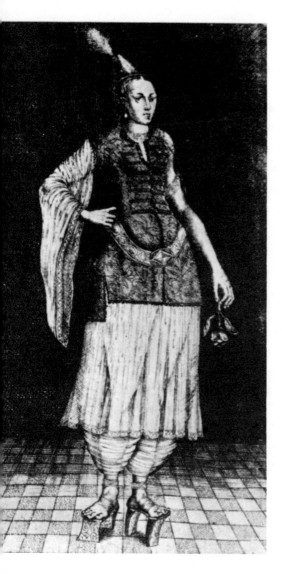 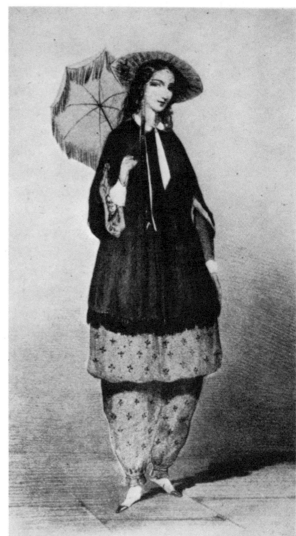

The American women who belonged to the sartorial liberation movement of the eighteen fifties ignored the free-flowing garments of antiquity and, lacking ideas of their own, settled for the dress of the very nation that had enslaved the descendants of the Greeks. Mrs. Amelia Bloomer's costume, a sensation on two continents, was closely modeled on what Turkish ladies wore long before the Pilgrims landed in the New World. The shapes of the two dresses are surprisingly alike, except that Mrs. Bloomer's sleeves, skirt and trousers were not transparent. Besides, her shoes had room for one toe only.

below the knees. Anxious to appear both modest and daring, she wore it over a pair of wide trousers, gathered above the ankles and made from the same material. She wore none of the then obligatory five to ten petticoats.

That same year she took the new costume to England, and soon women in bloomers were seen not only in London but as far as Scotland and Ireland. However, the "Turkish" trousers and "Syrian" dresses, as they were called abroad, never caught on because "the wearers were not sufficiently nerved to withstand for any length of time the persecuting curiosity excited by the trans-atlantic garb."

In the New World, that heretical contrivance, bloomers, fared worse. "I never believed in total depravity until I wore the reform dress in New York," wrote Maria M. Jones, another pioneering woman.[74] On the street, trousered women had to face moral and physical assault. Youngsters found in them an ideal target for snowballs and, in the warm season, for apple cores. Adults, not wanting to be left out, pelted them with verbal abuse. Even clergymen could be distinctly heard in the chorus of insulting voices. Women wearing the new dress were unceremoniously thrown out of churches and told that their attire would not be tolerated in places of worship or lecture halls.

Ironically, one of the arguments advanced in favor of reform dress by its addicts was its decorousness. It concealed the legs to perfection, which was not the case with the hoopskirts of the time. Mrs. Jones pitied the fashionable female who "frantically grasping her skirts in front with one hand, with the other lifts hoops and all behind her, and tiptoes across the street, with her clothing in the rear at an altitude of which she has no conception, and revealing, not only feet and ankles, but even limbs, to an extent which a neatly-clad Bloomer would blush to think of."[75] Physicians, who might have been expected to be on the side of reason, or at least to welcome a more hygienic female dress, lacked the courage to support the cause of the reformers. Unable to produce any sound argument against bifurcated skirts, they contented themselves with joining the-mob's laughter. "The idea of females wearing trousers," wrote *The Medical Times,* "may be scouted as ridiculous."

Mrs. Maria M. Jones, a prominent avant-gardeuse of dress reform, had to endure the wrath of her compatriotes who considered her trousers indecent.

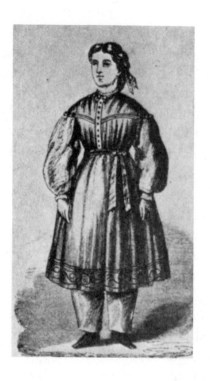

Mrs. Smith wore her costume for seven years, attending in it Washington's most elegant dinner parties. When, however, waitresses and vaudeville performers began to appear in trousers, their demise seemed inevitable. Mary E. Tillotson who published—in improved spelling—a history of the first thirty-five years of the reform movement in the United States, gave some reasons for its failure. "Among staid matrons hailing this reform as a saviour from dizeaz caused by labor under unnatural bodily burdens, many assumed the costume from love of novelty and in the hope that fashon would concur; ov cours a little ridicule redily restored the perilous petticoats ov such as these. Feeble ones groing strong in its use, and having minds to perceeve the revival ov all faculties, valued it highly; yet frends and pozishon tempted many ov the thautful to return, tho reluctantly. One whom I knu had her old shakles repaired for another slavery, a full year before she could bring her conshence to the test of violating all the best convictshons ov her being. Thus did thousands—thus do tha now—warp soul and body into the noose tha know is dezined to consume the effishency that would cultivate and manifest individual power and choice. Appaling times loom over humanity when so nearly all dare not enact known rite."[76] The collapse of the American dress reform movement was utter and complete.

Not for another two generations did fizical helth thru dress come true. Fainting females were the order of the day, and tubercular heroines ruled the literary stage; the adulation of the physically handicapped woman was general. "No girl in the physiology class had so small a waist," confessed one Miss Grace Greenwood; "I had occasional fainting fits, which rendered me interesting. For these and the ugly pain in the side, the cough and palpitations, physicians were called in. If they *thought* corsets, they did not mention them. Doctors were delicate in those days. Not knowing what to do, they bled me."[77]

Corset diseases—"ranging from haemorrhoids to cancer"—continued to plague fashionable women. Those who tried to improve their health through exercise, were severely censored. *"What has the average girl to do with a gymnasium?"* italicized the author of a book against rational clothes. "Sweeping and scrubbing a floor and dusting out a room, is infinitely more beneficial and useful than going to a sanctified room to turn somersaults."[78] The sanctified room was, however, indispensable; female exercises, being considered a most intimate body performance, had to be protected from the eye of man. Those who disdained the secrecy of four walls, exercised fully corseted, even though the hazards from splitting steel stays were well known. The only country that took exception to lacing was Russia where female students were forbidden to wear corsets.[79]

Incidentally, the use of knickers, "rationals," and "trowsers" helped to make people aware of the mechanics of dress. Yet one basic question remained unanswered; when at length the rebellious women worked up enough courage to discard the corset that had served seven generations, they realized with dismay that when it came to the problem of how to attach their improved dress to the body, the female torso was a poor substitute for the corset. Those who fastened their skirts around the hips soon discovered the disadvantage of this system. Skirts and petticoats were still unbelievably bulky, and the pressure of the waistband was only slightly less disagreeable than the pressure of the stays. The idea of suspending a dress from the shoulders proved equally impractical because of its excessive heaviness. (One Mrs. Parkins Gilman asserted that women have short legs because of the weight of clothing they have carried for so many centuries.) Speculation ensued, and schools of thought were founded on every new device for hanging dress on the peg that was the rediscovered human body. Moreover, since people were accustomed to the wasp waist with its rigorous division between the body's upper and lower part, they thought the new garments which restored anatomical unity unspeakably funny. When all was said and done, and every experiment had ended in disappointment, the plain fact emerged that in A.D. 1900, despite the examples of history, or for that matter, of contemporary oriental costume, people were ignorant of the principles of clothes construction.

Abroad, the dress revolt was fought by men who were, however, less interested in the shape of clothes than in their hygienic qualities. In Germany, the country that led the movement, the names

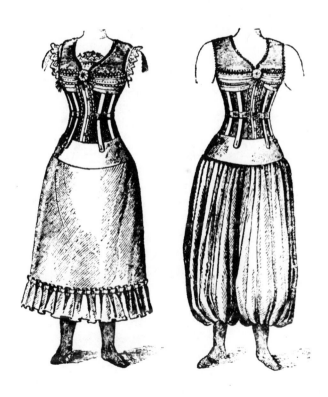

These supposedly wholesome garments, designed by a physician who took an active part in the women's reform movement, do not cast a favorable light upon the medical profession. But then, an uncorseted woman was a bawdy woman even in a doctor's eyes. From Dr. Spener's Die jetzige Frauenkleidung.

of pioneers such as Jäger, Lahmann, and Kneipp were household words. Each had his own theories and advocated what *he* believed to be the most hygienic clothing material. Lahmann and Kneipp sponsored cotton and linen respectively. Jäger recommended wool only; fearless of alliteration, he coined *Wer weise wählt Wolle*, the wise choose wool. His arguments were ingenious, his industry prodigious.

By far the most imaginative of the trio, Jäger had discovered the

184

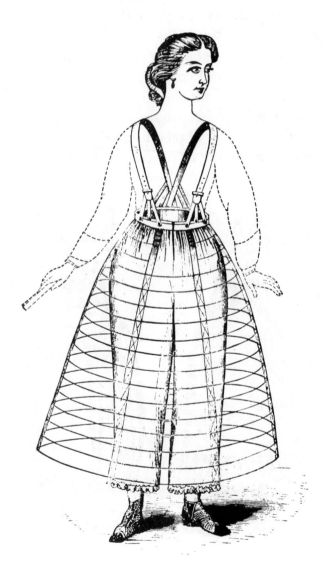

The efforts of the dress reformers were rewarded by the discovery of suspenders. Mrs. Jones joyously commented on the contraption: "I had overcome every obstacle but the support of the skirt; that, I was convinced, was insurmountable, when suddenly, by the inventive genius of a dear friend, the vexed problem was triumphantly solved, and practically demonstrated beyond the possibility of a doubt." From Maria M. Jones, Woman's Dress; its Moral and Physical Relations.

physical source of our emotions in some subtle essences contained in, and emitted by, our body. These essences, he maintained, were exhaled by mouth, nose, and skin, and *by the brain* as well, "as I have proved by experiment."[80] He divided body exhalations into salutary fragrant and noxious malodorous ones, and regarded the sexual instinct chiefly an olfactory matter. To follow his line of reasoning, a short digression on smell is in order.

Any healthy, clean person produces a number of different odors, not counting those of secretions and excretions. This is only as it should be for there is nothing wrong with giving off or being able to perceive a smell. Alexander the Great, Plutarch reports, exhaled so sweet an odor that his garments seemed to be soaked with aromatic perfumes. Physicians and psychologists proved this phenomenon to be true; "the recorded cases," wrote Ellis, "are very numerous in which persons have exhaled from their skin—sometimes in a very pronounced degree—the odors of plants and flowers, of violets, of roses, of pineapple, of vanilla." The Song of Songs is redolent of human perfume; the lovers' cheeks smell of herbs, their breasts of spices, their breath of apples. Men have been known to fall in love with the fragrance of a woman's body. Oriental potentates, forever vexed with the problem of choosing from their harem a daily companion, let their women exercise or race to make them perspire. The garments were then brought to them, and *she* was chosen who flattered their nostrils most. For another example, the exchange of garments among lovers, customary in past times, was motivated by their desire to retain each other's exhalations.

Again, the odor of sanctity that emanates from the body of a holy person is anything but a metaphor. It is due to abnormal nervous conditions, and is most noticeable at the hour of death. Odors act as powerful stimulants to the entire nervous system, and sensations of smell are known to induce the strongest emotions. Even the odors of flowers, exhaled during the reproductive period of the plant, are of a sexual character. Today's commercially available scents seem to lack this quality; many a woman has found to her chagrin that the purchase of a perfume with a name invoking venery fell short of helping bed her man. A few dabs behind her ear do not do the trick. What she needs is a good soaking. In biblical times such conditioning preceded a concubine's debut. "When every maid's turn was come to go in to the king Ahasuerus, after that she had been twelve months, according to the manner of the women, (for so were the days of their purifications accomplished, *to wit,* six months with oil of myrrh, and six months with sweet odors, and with *other* things for the purifying of the women)" (Esther, 2:12). This veritable marinade was not intended to blot out her natural smells but, on the contrary, to release and amplify them.

Only in our civilization of evil-smelling cities and landscapes has the word odor taken on the meaning of stench. To us, body odor means bad odor. The notion is by no means unjustified since our gamy smell is the result of a heavy meat diet. The last sweet-smelling American was Walt Whitman—if we can trust the word of his contemporaries.

To get back to Jäger and his startling insights into woolliness— his minute observations on the delicate relationship between the body and its coverings caught the imagination of the Teutonic mind right at the time when American women were wrestling with mere

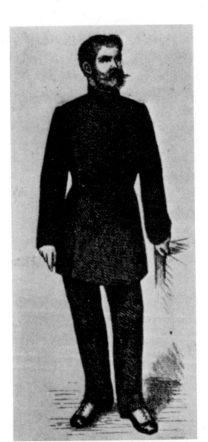

Dr. Gustav Jäger, wearing the reform dress he designed in 1880.

technical and aesthetic problems of dress. In dealing with smelly clothes, Jäger's merit and ensuing fame rest less on his discoveries than on his correct assessment of a reformer's business opportunities. In order to balance body odors and human emotions, he designed his Woollen System of Dress. He taught, and proved to the satisfaction of his countrymen, that woollen clothing (as long as it is not cleaned) retains those pleasant Alexandrinian emanations of the body that "induce a sense of vigor and sound health." Besides, woollen clothing, he maintained, permits the complete evaporation of the "noxious" essences.[81]

His view on corsets was no less original. Women's mistake, he pointed out, consisted not in wearing corsets but in choosing the wrong kind of material for them. Woollen corsets were of course the answer. A zoologist by profession, Jäger could not help being prejudiced in favor of animal fibers. Moreover, he belonged to a generation steeped in the study of classical writings and probably was well aware that the ancient Romans attributed magical virtues to wool. Wool, they believed, warded off evil forces. Wool symbolized purity—vestal virgins wore woollen garments only. Once Jäger had made up his mind to dress German womanhood in virgin wool, he began to attack every other material as noisome. "I have to declare war," he wrote, "against such cherished finery as silk dresses, white petticoats, linen stays, cotton and silk stockings, and white, starched dresses, which enclose the whole body like a glass cover. Chemise, stockings, drawers, petticoats, and stays should all be made of pure, animal wool. These, with a dress of pure woollen stuff, closing well round the throat, and having a double woollen lining at the chest and downwards, should be the winter and summer wear of women . . . "[82]

Men were not forgotten. The cut of Jäger's male costume was adapted from the soldier's uniform and represented an extreme case of the tubular style. He had hoped that it might become the German National Costume, but public opinion did not support him. His power of persuasion was not matched by any aesthetic sense. Nevertheless, his wares, which included woollen hats and boots and even woollen bedclothes, were sold everywhere, and his American catalog, *Dr. Jäger's Sanitary Woollen System of Dress*, testifies to

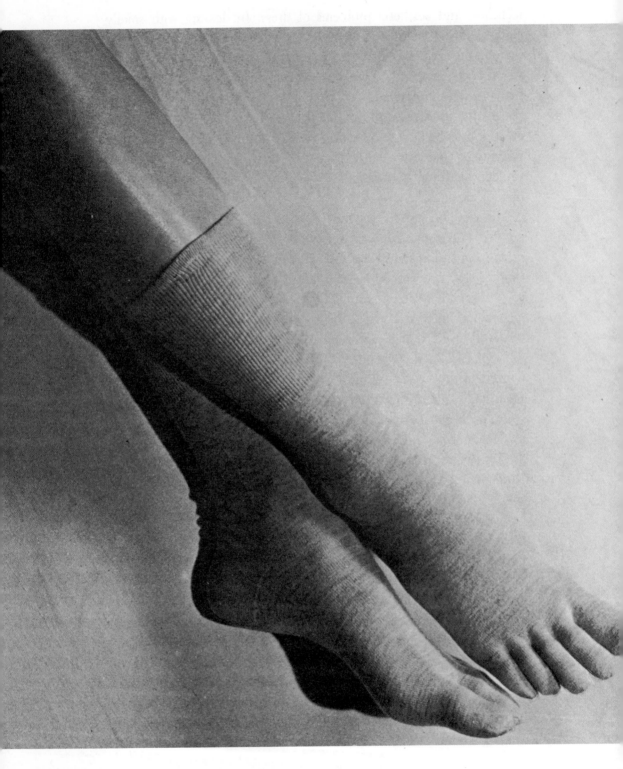

Stockings are as much responsible for deforming our feet as are shoes. Not so the digital socks, designed and manufactured by Gustav Jäger, that once were sold throughout the United States. Despite their woolliness, they are also esthetically superior to our inarticulate stockings. (Courtesy, The Metropolitan Museum of Art, New York)

his business acumen as a public relations man. Besides, his writings are studded with precious if old-fashioned advice. The wet body, he explained, should not be dried. "The wearer of the Sanitary Woollen Clothes must take pattern from the woollen-coated animal, which does not throw off its clothing, go into cold water, dry itself, and then resume its dry clothes, but goes, coat and all, into the water."[83] Again, "the wetting of the underclothing will be found a capital substitute for the refreshment of a bath when the bath cannot be had."[84] But the passage of time has dampened Jäger's words, his doctrine has acquired a moldy smell. His suggestion to wear a shirt for six or eight weeks between launderings has lost its appeal even for the thrifty.

The twentieth century saw the end of the reform movement. The last of the reform clothes, timid compromises with the haute-couture, were mostly on the dowdy side. The few women who had the nerve to wear unconventional garments are now forgotten, perhaps with the exception of Isadora Duncan, idolized by the Germans as the Holy Isadora. A shrewd provincial genius, she captured the world and its great men less by her posturing and preaching than by her courage to abjure the fashions of the day. Of generous proportions, running to corpulence, she used to swathe her figure in the thick folds of what was thought to be the costume of an Athenian matron. Such boldness is the stuff reformers are made of, yet aside from upholding her own costume as an example to her admirers, she actually never advocated any specific dress. Although she did urge the mayor of New York to put schoolchildren into uniforms, she only suggested a custom that she may have observed in foreign countries.

Once, musing on her turbulent life, she said that her real contribution to the world at large consisted in freeing women from the corset. But this was a beautiful illusion. What brought about the corset's disappearance was the necessity of conserving steel for armaments. One Mrs. Nicholas Longworth is credited with having decided that corsets were non-essential for her fellow women. Subsequently, a member of the War Industries Board revealed that the American women's sacrifice released 28,000 tons of steel during World War I, enough to build two battleships.

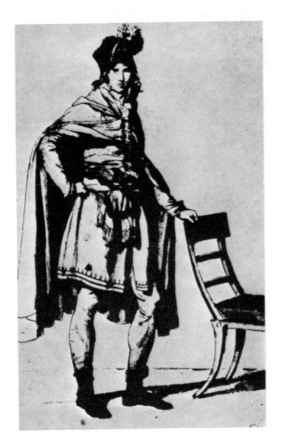

David's design for a French National Costume, made at Napoleon's request, was never carried out.

Coercive dress reform on a nationwide scale, which failed in France under Napoleon, succeeded in Turkey in our time. The cultural metamorphosis of Turkey is worth recalling because it demonstrates how dress and dress habits of a nation can be radically altered by the will of a single man. Kemal Pasha, later called Atatürk, the founder of modern Turkey, had firmly convinced himself that the only way to bring his country to the bosom of Western nations (97 percent of Turkey lies in Asia), was to erase her cultural heritage. Thus, to make the old literature inaccessible to the young, he substituted the Roman alphabet for Arabic writing; he banned many religious customs; he cajoled his countrymen into accepting Western art and architecture; he outlawed the status-imbued traditional costume as part of his efforts toward democratization in general, and Turkish women's emancipation in particular.

The introduction of Western-style clothing was but the finishing touch to his reform of all Turkish life.

In a way, Atatürk's dress reform was reform in reverse since some of the old costumes were in many respects superior to Western industrial dress. Surely, Mrs. Bloomer and her disciples would have been happy to swap clothes with Turkish women. But it was the trite and commonplace that suited the dictator's ideas best. "We shall wear shoes and boots," he ranted rapturously before the national assembly (bad footwear always heads the list of stratagems to inflict progress and punishment on mankind); "we shall wear trousers, shirts, waist-coats, collars, neckties; we'll have a headcovering with a brim, more precisely, we'll have a hat. We shall wear redingotes, jackets, dinner jackets and tail coats," and, he added angrily, "only idiots would hesitate to do so."[85] Sure enough, there were some who would rather die than submit to what they regarded an infamy. And die they did. After a few dozen dissenters had been hanged, the dress reform proceeded as smoothly as could be expected with the worst hat shortage in history. If memory serves, in the fall of 1925 Istanbul's streets presented a singular spectacle. Students' caps of German fighting fraternities, jockey caps, baby bonnets and tea cosies—I even spotted a few women's hats—adorned sad and beautiful faces with bushy brows and patriarchal beards. This vaudeville, remembered as "la crise des chapeaux" marked the triumphant arrival of Western culture.

In the old Othman empire, headgear, not clothes, made the man. To make a new start, Atatürk had to wipe out that most deeply engrained sartorial symbol of inequality, traditional headcoverings. Anybody who wants to form an idea of their variety has only to visit one of the magnificent cypress groves that proclaim the site of a Turkish cemetery from afar. The funereal trees shelter an outdoor museum that must warm a costumier's heart. Since the Koran does not permit the human figure in art, the Turks decorated their tombs with a stone replica of the dead man's headgear. The top of the vertical column that marks a grave—a kind of private dolmen —terminates in a stone bonnet minus a head. According to the man's rank it variously represents a finely chiseled turban, a dervish's cowl, a janizary's fez, or any of the assorted lids of a head-

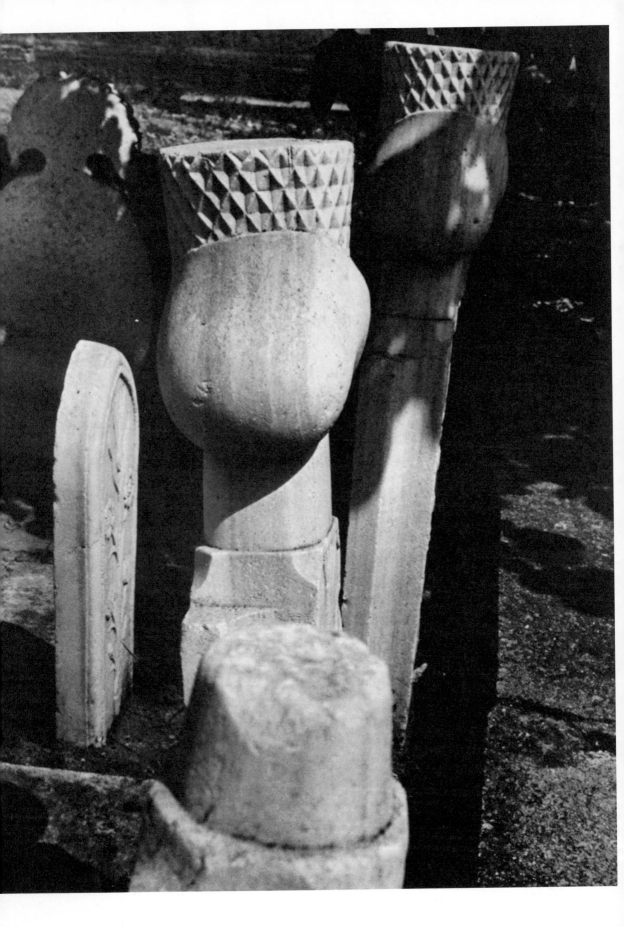

gear-conscious society. A stone turban set at a rakish angle does not memorialize a dandy but indicates that the man died by hanging. The tops of women's grave markers are bare; a flowery garland in bas relief snaking up the stele expresses her essentially forgettable station in life. These petrified fragments of the old Turkish costume are disappearing fast. Land speculators are encroaching on the sacred groves, and the ancient tombstones are discarded to make room for new ones, styled in the tradition of the Père Lachaise, with oval sepia photographs under glass that recall the deceased's likeness.

On the opposite end of the Asian continent, in Japan, a national dress reform, motivated by much the same considerations as the Turkish one, was undertaken about one hundred years ago. It was of the first magnitude, intended to recast a wardrobe for more than thirty million people. It, too, was the by-product of a larger upheaval, the transformation of Japan into a modern nation, or, to put it less grandly, the submission of an old culture to Western ideas and ideals, traditionally scorned by Orientals. It so happens that Japanese classical costume represents an achievement unmatched since ancient Greece. Despite some inconsistencies and irrationalities (e.g. the authentic kimono is taken apart every time it is cleaned), it would seem to have its place in the future as much as it had in the past. If simplicity, tempered by elegance, is the recognized aim of apparel, Japanese costume contains enough germinative ideas to keep us well supplied for centuries to come. So far it has hardly found its due.

To think that a garment was so ingeniously constructed that it would fit anybody! For, as in classical antiquity, neither clothes nor shoes were tailored. Footwear came in two sizes only: large for men and small for women. (Traditional footwear—the stilted wooden clogs favored by young and old alike—still does.) Considering as they did healthy feet indispensable for their well-being, the Japanese were anxious to assure their toes' free movement. Instead of shutting them off in shoes, they wore dozens of different types of open sandals.

The advantages resulting from the absence of dress and shoe sizes are too obvious to be discussed—with one exception: When

urbaned tombstones in a Turkish cemetery.

*The supreme ugliness of some of Western man's clothes is summarized
in this nineteenth-century drawing from a Japanese dictionary.*

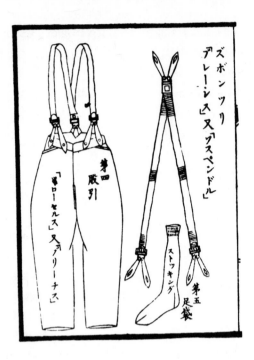

traveling in Japan there is no need to lug around one's own clothes.
Just as we take it for granted that sheets and towels are provided
by a hotel (a convenience of relatively recent date), a genuine
Japanese inn supplies its guests with a complete wardrobe during
their stay. It consists of a daily laundered light gown for indoors,
a padded outer garment for cold weather, a straw hat and oiled-
paper umbrella, slippers, sandals, and clogs of every description.
The tourist who wants to sample old-fashioned comfort still finds
Japan the only place on earth where he can travel lightly. He can
roam the country minus the sort of baggage that with us often
comes close to being the very motivation for a journey.

In the eighteen-seventies all these and many more built-in advantages of their costume the Japanese were asked to abandon in
favor of alien amenities and, eager as they were to rise from their
knees to their feet, actually and metaphorically, they went about
their conversion with commendable dispatch. As always, the introduction of bad footwear is the first step toward westernizing man.
Instead of seizing this opportunity to revolutionize shoe design—
and thereby producing shoes for their undeformed feet—the
Japanese satisfied themselves with copying Western shoes. The

government took the lead. To complement the new military uniform, boots were made on foreign lasts. As one historian recalls, "not a single Japanese foot could be found to fit them. They were thrown away." Although the Japanese have long become reconciled to shoes, they draw the line at traditional costume; they never wear shoes with kimono. The foreign woman in kimono and high-heeled shoes makes them wince.

Western clothes hardly made a better start. Adequate as they proved for office and workshop, they turned out to be unsuitable to the furnitureless Japanese house where one sits on the floor. They had one good point; compared to Japanese costume they were cheap. Alas, people soon discovered to their dismay that they were a poor investment since their usefulness was short-lived. For reasons not immediately transparent, they had to be discarded long before

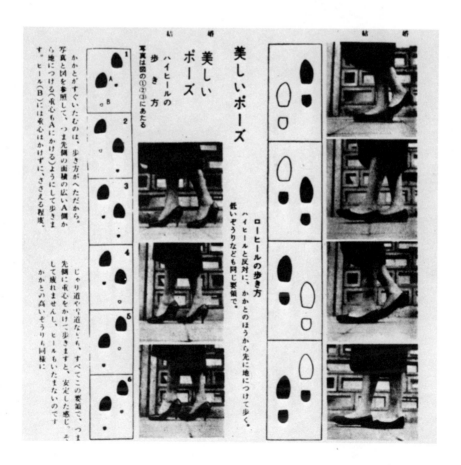

More than hundred years after Western dress was introduced to Japan, part of it still baffles the wearer. A page from a modern etiquette book illustrates how women learn to walk in Western shoes. For some of them lifting their feet is more difficult than learning a new dance step is to us.

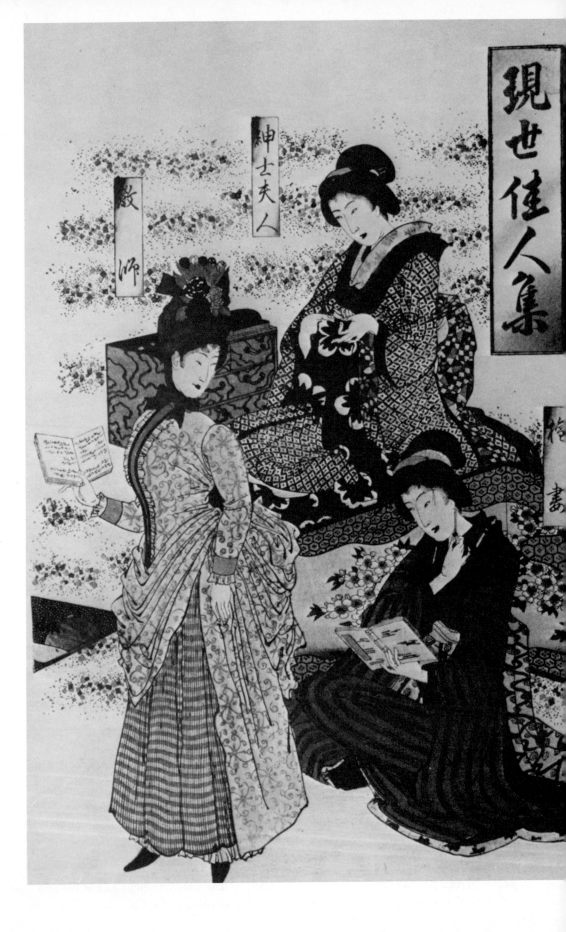

they wore out. A dress which elicited admiration today, made one the laughingstock tomorrow. Clearly, foreign clothes were inferior to native ones. The unceasing change in styles was just another proof of Western man's notorious insecurity in all matters of taste.

As soon as the novelty of crinolines and bonnets, of jackets, trousers and felt hats had worn off, some of the old costumes returned to popularity. In fact, they were increasingly worn in preference to, and in protest against, foreign dress. In the end patriotism gave way to conformity; a compromise was reached by adopting the new and retaining the old. Traditional garments were given a new lease on life by being promoted to formal and festive wear. Thus, the coexistence of oriental and Western dress was accepted by all and contributed to no small degree to the nation's cultural schizophrenia that is the delight of the Japanophile.

The conversion of the rest of the world to Western dress encountered little resistence. The last of the self-appointed reformers, the missionary, has long been on the wane. But during the nineteenth century, the heyday of his reign, he practiced cultural rape with gusto and impunity. Insensitive to the better things in life, he championed Victorian morality with distasteful zeal. By projecting his own fear and hatred of the human body into and beyond his hapless community, he was able to strike at the people's most vulnerable spot, their self-respect, and to force them into garments that were "injurious to their health, degrading to their dignity." Conditions in a Tonga village in 1894 can be gleaned from the report by a former governor: " . . . it was punishable by fine and imprisonment to wear native clothing; punishable by fine and imprisonment to wear long hair or a garland of flowers; punishable by fine and imprisonment to wrestle or to play ball; punishable by fine and imprisonment to build a native-fashioned house; punishable not to wear shirt and trousers, and in certain localities coat and shoes also . . . "[86] It seems doubtful that a roasted missionary ever yielded an enjoyable meal.

Japanese school mistress in Western dress with bustle.
Anonymous nineteenth-century woodcut.
(Courtesy, Print Collection, New York Public Library)

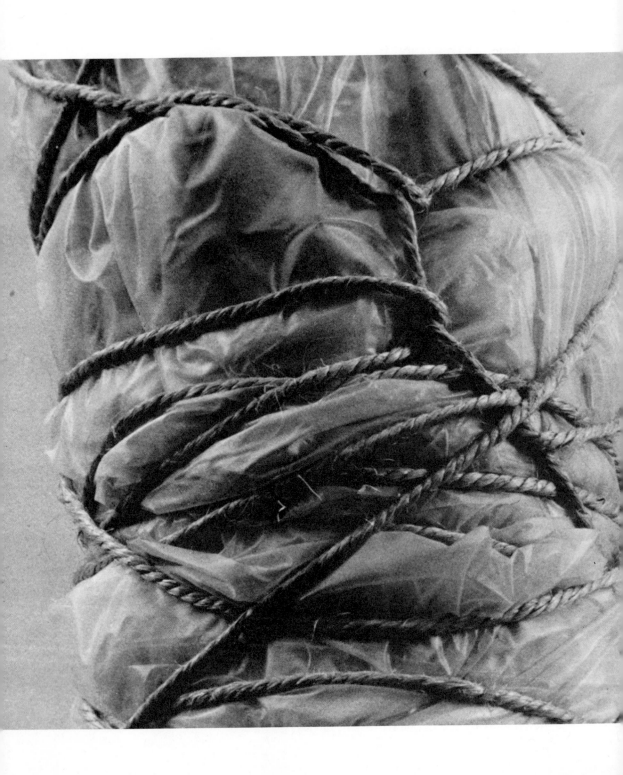

Sartoriasis, the enjoyment of discomfort

In his *Anatomy of Melancholy* (1624), Burton observed that "the greatest provocations of lust are from our apparel."[87] Psychologists not only proved him correct but confirmed the belief that these provocations have been consciously sought, except perhaps in our time when the pleasures derived from the embrace of dress are practically unknown. Our ignorance—or indifference—can be laid to lack of curiosity and imagination on the part of both the makers and the wearers of clothes and, more generally, to the fact that of all races ours is the least alert in matters of sensuality.

The intoxication obtained from wearing certain articles of clothing can be as powerful as that induced by a drug. The effects of this sartorial self-indulgence run the gamut from innocent fantasies to physical and mental disorders that are rarely discussed or avowed. The music historian Kalbeck refers to the tame sort of stimulation when he tells us about a young woman who exclaimed at a concert: "One enjoys music twice as much *décolletée!*" The assault of symphonic sound, not just upon the eardrums but upon those parts of the skin that women traditionally exhibit at social gatherings, produced a multiple thrill, lasciviousness of the heart, the word to be understood in its original sense.

Torso," by Christo.

A similar kind of lustful sensation, equally chaste and more than a trifle puerile, was experienced by the last German emperor, Wilhelm II, when attending performances of *The Flying Dutchman* dressed in the uniform of an admiral. This was an ingenious ruse for intensifying his empathy to the bubbly score and, in a more subtle way, identifying himself, if on a much higher echelon, with the protagonist of the opera.

The whole point about dress, Eric Gill once remarked, is that it fits a person mentally rather than physically. Yet has there ever been a psychiatrist known to employ sartorial therapy, that is, to prescribe *disguises* for his patients, to lessen their real or imagined sufferings? To be sure, some people on their flight from the banality of everyday life have sought the psychic shelter of fancy dress of their own account. The original dropout, the bluestocking of the Victorian era, was one of them. Before retiring to her Turkish corner with an unexpurgated copy of *The One Thousand and One Nights*, she slipped into pantaloons and pantouffles that transported her into agreeable reveries. Although the titillations of the printed page need not be minimized, her change of clothes played the larger part in her fantasies. It was the epidermal contact with a costume symbolizing erotic savoir-faire that triggered her emotional escape from the workaday world. (This ever-present impulse to romantically disguise oneself has found a regular outlet only in our time. In recent years, harem costumes of every erotomanic nuance have been available at clothing stores to be worn not only in the intimacy of bedroom and boudoir but sometimes in the ignominious blaze of lights at a supermarket.)

Ideally, there is nothing like strange clothes to break down the barriers that imprison our imagination. On the stage costume is all important. It creates and sustains illusions incomparably more powerful than those derived from scenery or the spoken word. Strip an actor of his legitimate costume, as has been done in productions where Caesar appeared in slacks or Hamlet in white tie, and you find that scenery can be dispensed with but not costume. Histrionics simply do not compensate for the lack of an appropriate masquerade. And although an actor does not expect his stage dress alone to bridge the gap of space and time that separates him from the historical or

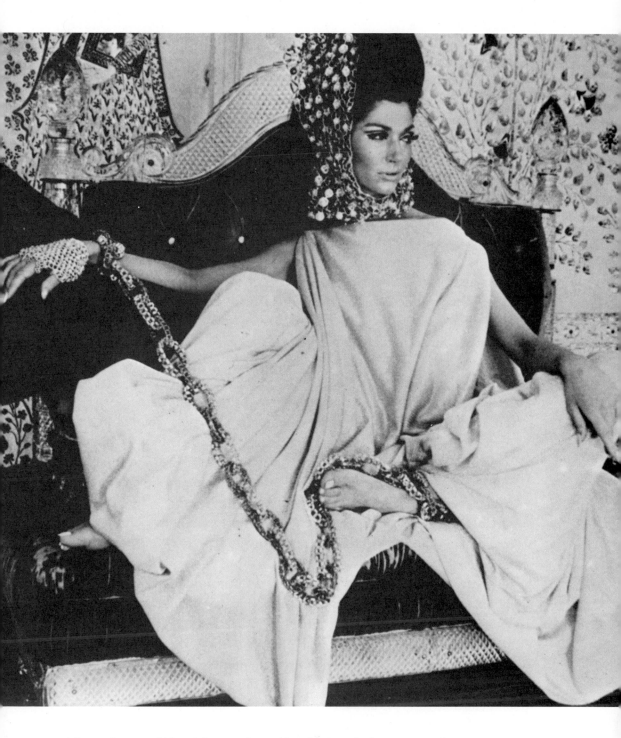

The modern would-be odalisque, chained hand to foot, finds erotic stimulation in enforced immobility. (Courtesy Vogue. Copyright © 1967 by The Condé Nast Publications, Inc.)

fictional character he impersonates, it enables him to surpass himself by forgetting his identity, if only for some precious moments.

Our bluestocking *qua* odalisque was far more methodical in her pursuit of pleasure than we might think. Chafing against ennui, immured in a world of ugliness, she craved for its antipodes, the fabled Orient. Her bogus harem costume was the perfect choice of travel outfit for her imaginary excursions. Moreover, fashionable literature just happened to cater to her needs. The Romantic School of the nineteenth century had spawned exoticism, a literary form concerned with what one of its practitioners called "the infinite of nostalgia." This sentimental attachment to more or less inaccessible countries was cultivated by a restless band of French and English poets and novelists rich in eccentricity ("I was born to live in the Orient," noted the teen-age Flaubert in his diary) some of whom tried—but never quite succeeded—to assuage their malaise through extended travels and sojourns in the Near East. To them, travel was as much a state of mind as a way of life. Travel was slow, and deliberately so. In order to educate their sensibilities, these men rejected the rôle of the spectator to assume that of a full participant. To further explore their emotional promptings, they voluntarily underwent *dépaysement*, the estrangement from one's country. This sometimes involved marrying, if only temporarily, a native woman, a pursuit of happiness no more frivolous or dishonorable than our national divorce game. It also meant wearing native dress, and observing native customs. Compared to our doltish standards of organized tourism the hardships and hazards involved were considerable. Occasionally, as in Byron's case, the adventure ended in death.

Exoticism and eroticism went hand in hand. "A love of the exotic," affirms Mario Praz, an eminent critic of romantic writings, "is usually an imaginative projection of sexual desire. This is quite clear in the cases of Gautier and Flaubert, whose dreams carried them into worlds of barbaric and Oriental antiquity, where the most unbridled desires can be indulged and the cruelest fantasies can take concrete form."[88] Dress, especially woman's, played a prominent part in these fantasies; one cannot help noticing that the writers waxed lyrical every time they described the disquieting splendor of female *toilettes*.

Flaubert's *Salammbô* is a case in point. Although the book was no great literary success, the heroine's wardrobe still wears well. One little number, a giant snake, tastefully coiled around her naked body—a mobile garment, so to speak—is timeless, never in fashion, never outmoded. Salammbô's more conventional coming-out dress, the one she wears in the first chapter of the novel, is no less a show stopper: "Her hair, powdered with violet dust, was gathered up into a tower in the manner of Canaanite maidens and added to her stature. Strands of pearls fell from her temples down to the corners of her mouth, a rosy half-open pomegranate. Her sleeveless black tunic was studded with red flowers and exposed her bare arms bedecked with diamonds. Between her ankles she wore a golden chain to regulate the length of her steps, and her dark cloak trailed

203

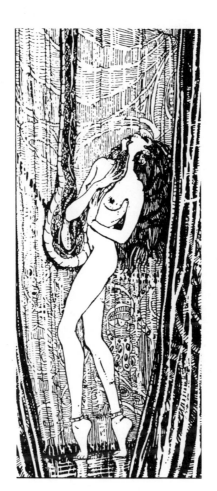

Detail from an illustration by Mahlon Blaine.
to Flaubert's Salammbô.

behind her, billowing with each step."

Clearly, Flaubert had shunned no expense for his literary chor-
eography; on the verbal level the design was impeccable—a mixture
of pathetic tenderness and awe. Yet fully to appreciate the nostalgic
quality of his sartorial inventions, we have to contrast them with
the numbingly drab kind of garments, male and female, worn in
his own day and environment. This is how he introduces Emma

Bovary: "Her neck rose from a white, turned-down collar. The two
black coils of her hair were so smooth that they seemed composed
of a single tress that separated in the middle of her forehead and
permitted only the end of her ears to be seen. At the back they
mingled in an abundant chignon." Her dress is not mentioned
except for two buttons of her bodice between which she carried,
"like a man," a tortoise-shell eyeglass.

To be sure, *Madame Bovary* belongs to the genre of the realistic
novel, where women perspire, men smell of tobacco, and the poor
(and middle-class) man's opera is the bed. It was the romantic,
exotic novel that discovered the charms of uncorseted women, and
with it the libertinism of oriental costume. Yet almost a century had
to pass before some of its principles were absorbed into Western
female clothes. The freedom of dress that we take for granted today
then existed only in the febrile minds of artists and writers.

On the whole, these literary improvisations paled before the true-
life stories of more enterprising men. The darling of the exoticists
was Gérard de Nerval, who embodied the perfect image of the romantic poet by committing suicide at the age of thirty-seven. Perhaps
the most uninhibited of those fantasts, he found "inexpressible satisfaction" in daydreams, usually assisted by liberal doses of hashish
and opium. Aware as he was that the Near Orient of the 1840s
might not live up to his expectations of sensual thrills—we have to
bear in mind that his favorite haunt, Othman Turkey, was culturally
much closer to Theodora's Byzantium than to the aseptic westernized country today's tourist sees through his car window—he nevertheless gave it a try, and in the course of events became a
conscientious and observant traveler.

Nerval's first impulse on visiting Turkey was to go native, not
only better to insinuate himself into the maelstrom of pleasures but

to shed the old Adam imprisoned in Western dress. He shaved his head, trimmed his beard in the Levantine fashion, and donned a turban and Turkish clothes "of such sure taste that the most discriminating eye could not detect the disguised European." This outfit, he admitted was far more than a ruse; it stood, a precious symbol for his spiritual metamorphosis. Wearing an exotic costume, he wrote, "made me feel that *I was changing the conditions of good and evil.*"[89] (Italics added.) His observation that life around him resembled "a perpetual opera ball where the guests were not allowed to drop their masks," is hardly profound, yet it conveyed the joy of one who until then had known colorful civilian clothes only from the stage or the mummified exhibits in museum vitrines.

Artists were, if anything, even more avid for relaxing their self-discipline than writers. In their surrender to the caresses of oriental and mock-oriental trappings they found—often without recourse to drink and drugs—gratification of their romantic leanings. "Are we ourselves at the end of what a more advanced civilization can produce?" wrote the young Delacroix in 1832 during a six-month sojourn in northern Morocco. "They [the Moroccans] are closer to nature in a thousand ways: in their clothes, in the form of their shoes. Hence beauty is linked to everything they do. In our corsets, our tight shoes, our ridiculous sheaths, we inspire pity."[90] On his return from Africa Delacroix continued to paint his monumental historical tableaux; it was left to an artist of sedentary habits, Matisse, to celebrate the beauty of uncorseted, barefoot women in his series of *Odalisques*.

Oriental dress stood for a way of life still untainted by contact with the infidel and, literally, unclean Westerner. The cleanliness that had gone out of Western life with the departure of the Moors from Spain was now being rediscovered as an adjunct to oriental dress by literati and artists, men reputed to be temperamentally inclined to side with St. Jerome, who praised the nuns for never letting water touch their bodies. Nerval, Gautier, Lamartine, pounced on the *hammam*, the Turkish bath. "Only the Turks," they claimed, "know how to bathe."

The bath—not, of course, the dreary performance that *we* call a bath but its time-honored classical concept—stands for unceasing

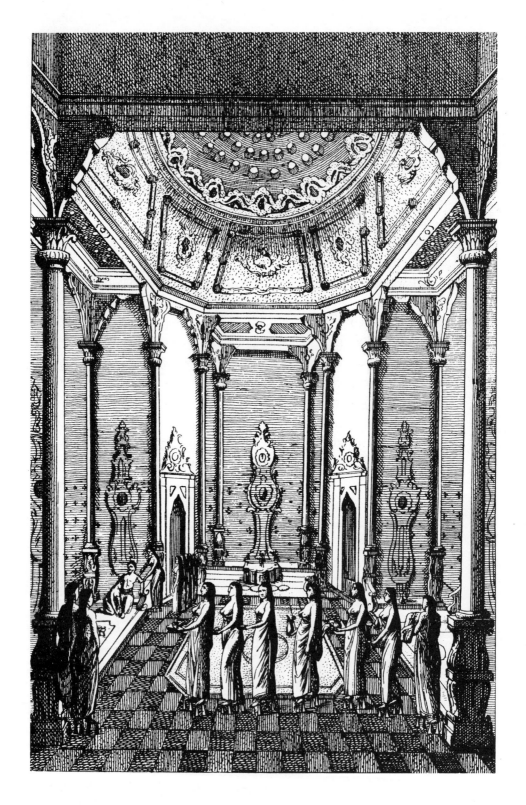

"The Sultan's bathroom." *Giulio Ferrario,* Il costume antico e moderno.

regeneration of the body. The daily use of facilities for swimming, sweating, and massage produces a physique of incomparably higher vitality than one that gets aired only during vacation time. More importantly, and quite apart from water therapy, bathing educates the sense of touch, a fact that disturbs people who shun the "voluptuous embrace of hot water." The relationship between bath and dress may not be obvious at first, yet one is probably justified in relating open pores to an open mind. Since nobody so far has connected a bathing culture with wearing apparel, this oversight shall be remedied herewith.

It is no coincidence that the nations who achieved a body culture through a highly developed bathing routine happen to be the very same who produced intelligently conceived forms of dress. The men and women who frequented the ancient thermae wore loose garments of the simplest shape. So did, and to a degree still do, Orientals, whereas Western nations with their hermetic clothes were throughout history (except in the Middle Ages) farthest removed from contact with water. Indeed, at the time when Western dress was at its most sumptuous, the bath had been consigned to oblivion. At Versailles, the very citadel of the Occident, people refused to have anything to do with bathing. The dukes and princes who occasionally dressed up in the flamboyant costume of Le Grand Turc, could bear each other's presence only thanks to generous dousings with perfume.

The limpid atmosphere of the Islamic bath provided a superb setting for social intercourse although, unlike the medieval European bath, it was not promiscuous. As early as in the eighteenth century it had been brought to the attention of the English public by the Right Honorable Lady Mary Wortley Montagu, the eccentric wife of Britain's ambassador to the Sublime Porte. Feminist, poet, medical pioneer, and indefatigable traveler, she is chiefly remembered for her spirited letters, which won her the admiration of Voltaire, Johnson, and the great of her day. Traveling as she did with a bodyguard of five hundred janizaries on journeys "not undertaken by any Christian since the time of the Greek emperors,"[91] she came across things unknown and unsuspected by her and her countrymen and recorded them with rare candor.

Like Nerval, whom she preceded by four generations, she adopted native clothes and dressed *alla turca*, although she entertained doubts about her disguise's effectiveness. On her first visit to a bath house, however, she happened to wear her ordinary travel outfit, a European costume. She had no intention of getting wet; indeed, she did not even take off her clothes. Despite her slightly patronizing attitude toward her hosts—two hundred women, stark naked, "only adorned by their beautiful hair"—she seems to have been well aware of looking a sight herself. "The lady," she wrote, "that seemed the most considerable among them entreated me to sit with her, and would fain have undressed me for the bath. I excused myself with difficulty. They being however so earnest in persuading me, I was at last forced to open my shirt, and shew them my stays, which satisfied them very well; for, I saw they believed I was locked up in that machine, and that it was not in my power to open it, which contrivance they attributed to my husband."[92]

This thwarted collision between Nereids and an armor-plated Englishwoman in Turkish waters (an underwater corset is shown on page 111) came as close to an allegory of Eastern and Western dress as fraternization would allow. What spoiled the idyll was *that machine*, which the Mussulwomen correctly interpreted as an outsize version of a chastity belt: It prevented the curious guest from being a woman among women.

A healthy respect for the human body: a preference for ample garments plus loose footwear, for houses unencumbered by furniture and knick-knack, was shared by such diverse, geographically and historically distant civilizations as classical antiquity, the Islamic world, and Japan (the two latter before their westernization). All were blessed with a mental climate where cleanliness was valued as a moral virtue, and ablutions figured among religious exercises. (In 1890, William James had this to say on our nonexistent desire for bathing: "We 'wash-up' and set ourselves right, at moments when our social selfconsciousness is awakened, in a manner toward which no strictly instinctive native prompting exists. But the standard of cleanliness, attained in this way is not likely to go beyond the mutual tolerance for one another of the members of the tribe and

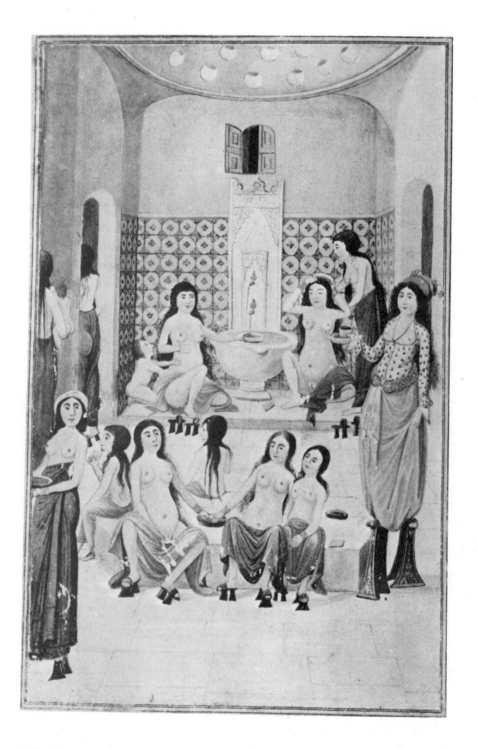

"The Women's Bath." From a manuscript of the *Zanan-nameh,* by Fazil
Yildiz 2824–73. (Courtesy, University Library, Istanbul).

hence may comprise a good deal of actual filth.")[93]

In the rivalry between antagonistic cultures, the basic motivations for or against body care are easily confused or misunderstood. While one nation treasures the bath as something akin to a sacrament, another sees in it an abomination. Similarly, the very same kind of dress is believed by some people to glorify the body, by others to defile it. We conveniently forget that the function of dress goes far beyond covering and adorning the body. Dress determines posture and movement; it animates or slows down its wearer. It influences the way people walk, run, squat, kneel, and sit, all of which reflect cultural traits. Not only that; each familiar gesture or posture is considered correct, each unfamiliar one undignified. When Melville spoke of people who "recline like voluptuous Orientals," he betrayed not only his own prejudice but also his fellow men's emotional inability to tolerate folkways other than their own. To us, reclining has always had orgiastic connotations. It conjures up bacchanalian banquets,

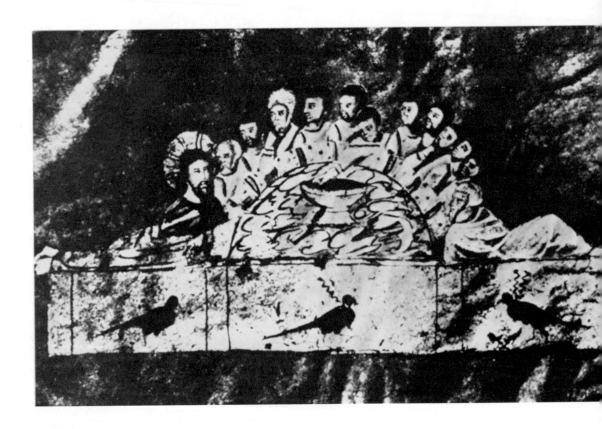

Last Supper. Painted on purple parchment.
Codex Rossanensis. *Sixth century.*

a form of entertainment as alien to us as a *bonne table*. To make Himself acceptable to us, that most blameless of Orientals, Jesus Christ, had to give up, posthumously, His way of dining in the reclining position. The legions of artists who portrayed the Last Supper had to help Him to a sitting position to keep us ignorant about His "voluptuous" table manners.

Melville probably never made a try at postural voluptuousness. For one thing, his clothes and furniture were not suitable; for another, he lacked the grace to enjoy himself. And so it is with us. Even if we should want to give reclining a chance, we would experience nothing more alarming than some slight discomfort—a cramp perhaps, an arm gone asleep—but no feelings even remotely sensuous.

Pleasant feelings, of a different kind and difficult to describe, are derived from extending our body by means of apparel, accessories, and sundry appendages: A trailing robe, a cape ballooning in the wind, a towering hairdo or a tall hat, a lorgnon, a pipe—all help to increase our tactile range, much as a pair of binoculars expands our field of vision. In a sense, these artificial excrescences take the place of animals' spines, spurs, horns, and antlers. (To lend a touch of ferocity to their battle dress, such dissimilar peoples as the Teutons and the Japanese actually grafted horns and antlers onto their helmets.)

Touching a thing, or a person, indirectly, that is, with an object held in one's hand, is called "double contact." It is supposed to produce sensations of heightened self-awareness, and there is no reason to doubt this. For instance, it is nearly impossible for a person to tickle himself with his fingers. However, he easily succeeds when using an extraneous object like a feather. An inanimate object such as a walking stick turns into a feeler and, through the hand's touch, becomes infused, as it were, with our life sap. In the old Japan, in the thick of battle, a warlord waved an *iron* fan to emphasize his orders. The military use of what we take to be an instrument of flirtation, appears somewhat less absurd when we remember that artists liked to portray a commander-in-chief on the battlefield with his drawn sword pointing to where the action is. Pointing a finger is unheroic—worse, indelicate. Hence the conductor's baton.

Today, the tactile sensations derived from dress, the undulations of pain and pleasure, are mostly forgotten or unsuspected. Although seduction by way of garments, ornaments, and scents lately is bandied about more than ever, autoeroticism is only beginning to come into its own. Psychologists, who have a proprietary interest in the subject, speak of skin- and muscle-eroticism, both of which apply to the clothed body as much as to the nude one. As a rule, however, only so-called wholesome aspects are discussed: the effects of heat and cold, of water and wind on muscles and skin—stimulations that are considered legitimate. Recommended, prescribed, and indulged in with moderation, they are thought to be eminently beneficial. Not so stimulation—a better word is perhaps titillation—connected with narcissistic and exhibitionistic pleasures.

Apart from constituting the body's outer envelope, the skin is the erogenic zone par excellence, the seat of touch, that most widely diffused and most fundamental of our senses. Love, said Mantegazza, is but a higher form of the sense of touch. Everbody knows from his own experience that some regions of the body's surface are more responsive to touch than others. Mouth, nipples, armpits, and, on a different sensory level, finger tips and toes, elbows and knees, even the palm of the hand and the sole of the foot, have been defined as areas "whose stimulation gives rise, directly or indirectly, to voluptuous sensations."[94] Although our skin cannot compete with the complex and specialized types of skin animals are invested with, it has nevertheless been identified as the most reliable source of our knowledge of the external world. The stimuli received can provoke exquisite sensations—particularly sexual ones. They are not necessarily caused by person-to-person contact but may ignite from the touch of inanimate objects such as garments and ornaments.

The pleasurable experience of stroking, or merely brushing against, silk, velvet or fur is largely ignored today; it is not quite clear what has changed or gone astray—our sense of touch or the quality of dress materials. Obviously, dress, that time-honored coating, even in its antisensual forms, plays on some of the focal points of the body. Our forebears did not always register agreeable feelings in connection with textiles or furs because these were often offset by a garment's unpleasant features. Such unpleasantness was usually

Corsets and hobbleskirts being temporarily out of fashion, those in need of physical restraint have to make do with arm and leg bands. (Courtesy Vogue *Copyright © 1970 by The Condé Nast Publications, Inc.)*

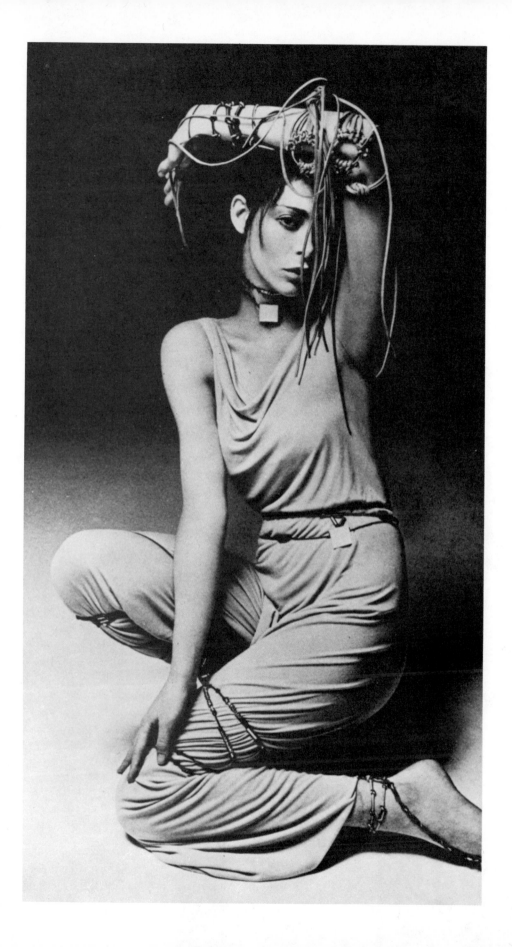

taken for granted; in fact, it was thought to be in the disciplinarian nature of dress. Conscious as most people were of the moral purpose of covering their nakedness, they may even have welcomed some degree of discomfort. The belief in the chastening power of uncomfortable dress, the moral itch, so to speak, was as deeply rooted in their minds as the belief that a cold climate stimulates the brain.

Still, uncomfortable dress has its compensations. The hair shirts of saints and sinners seem to have been far from unbearable. Ever since it was discovered that wild honey and locusts (toasted to a

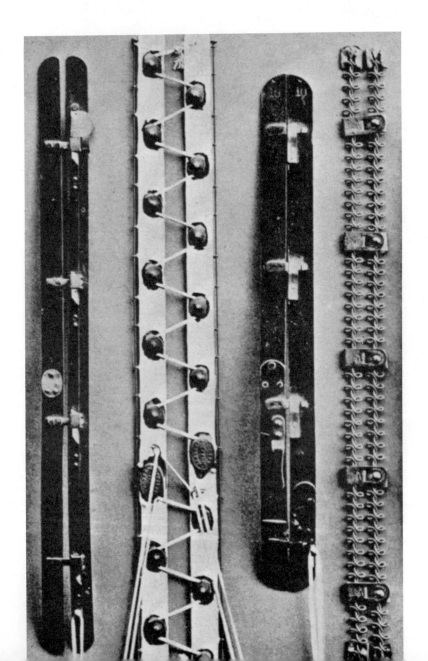

Nineteenth-century corset hardware. From Libron and Clouzot, Le corset dans l'art et les moeurs.

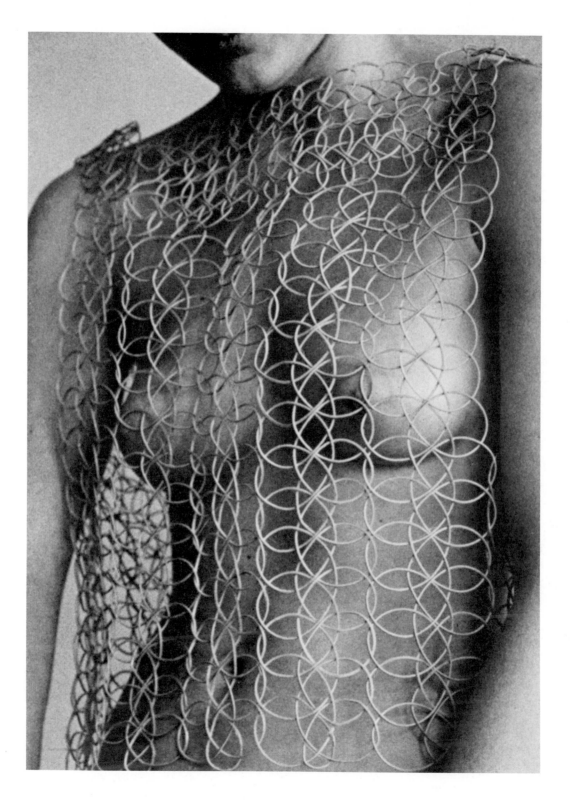

*This Japanese shirt, made of braided bamboo, is sold
in shops that specialize in religious articles.*

crisp) do not make a starvation diet but are, on the contrary, a gourmet's delight, penitential garments have been regarded with suspicion. A professional ascetic's life of attrition was not without its rewards. "Camlet, hair cloth, and articles of wool or hair," observed one writer on the murkier aspects of eroticism, "with which pious individuals have clothed themselves, have often contributed, with certain disciplines, to induce incontinence."[95] No matter; today we know on good authority that St. John the Baptist wore nothing itchier than a camel's hair coat.

Clothes as tools of moral and physical self-gratification have a long history. Elizabethans defended their right to wear a millstone of starched lace around their necks. The double-edged ruff resembled nothing so much as a stylized Chinese *cangue*, the portable wooden pillory carried by offenders convicted of petty crimes. Both fitted tightly around the neck, but unlike the lacy European version, the heavy—from forty to sixty pounds—Chinese one was also worn at night. A less remote example of this kind of chafing choker is the stiff shirt collar. It triumphed in the Hoover era when a gentleman deprived of his high collar felt spiritually naked.

Prodigious sources of skin and muscle sensations are tapped by those exceedingly narrow waistbands, belts, and bodices that reappear with regularity on the fashionable scene. At one time or another, these instruments of self-torture were essential parts of our wardrobe. The pressure they exert on the body is a hindrance to

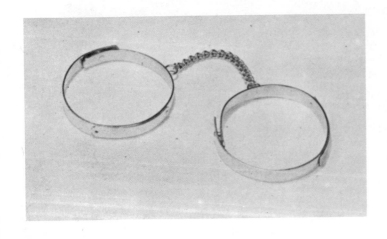

Handcuff jewelry, 1946. (Courtesy, Charm magazine)

Opposite: In our day the tonic effect of cutaneous stimulation is sought by means of tight-fitting belts, arm bands, straps and lacings, that produce a perpetual, albeit impersonal caress.
(Courtesy Vogue. *Copyright © 1970 by The Condé Nast Publications, Inc.*

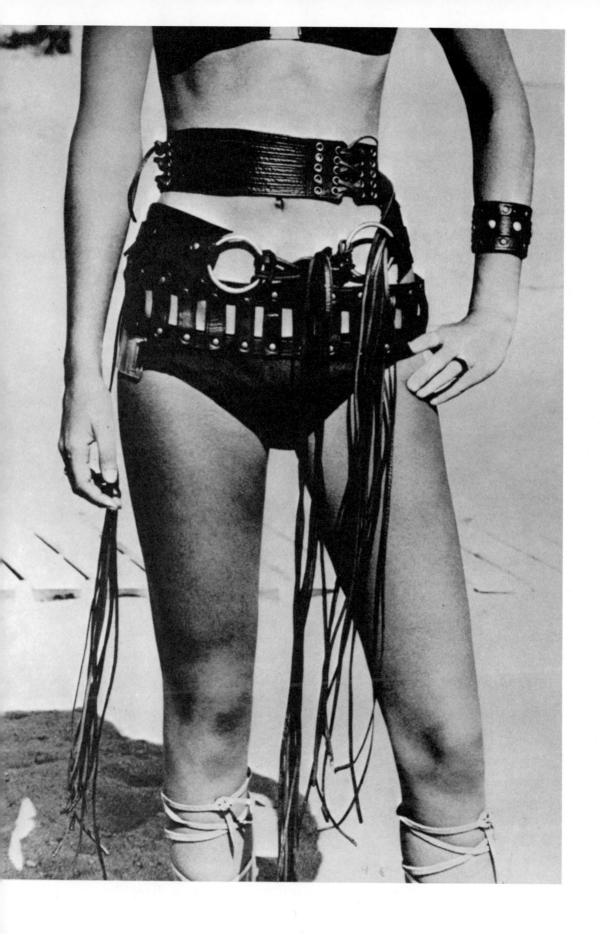

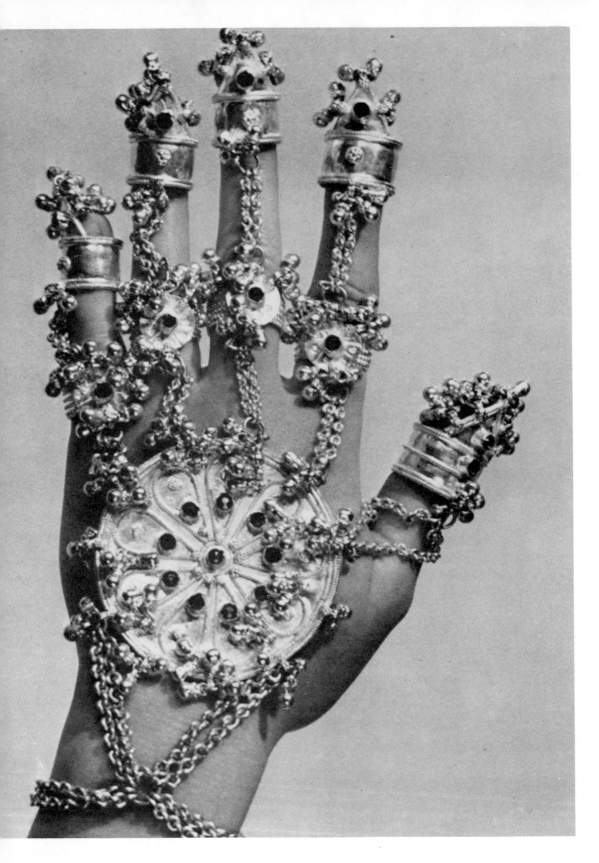

This Indian ornament, a stylized glove, consists of rings and chainlets that imprison the hand. Ahmedabad, Guharat States. (Courtesy, Musée de l'Homme, Paris)

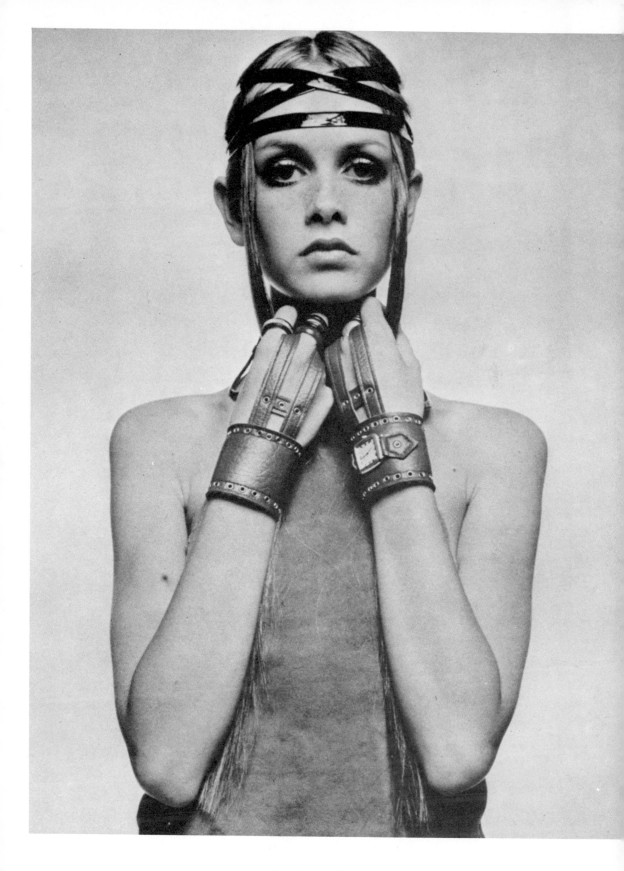

*Leather handstraps, 1967. (Courtesy Vogue.
Copyright ⓒ 1967 by The Condé Nast Publications, Inc.)*

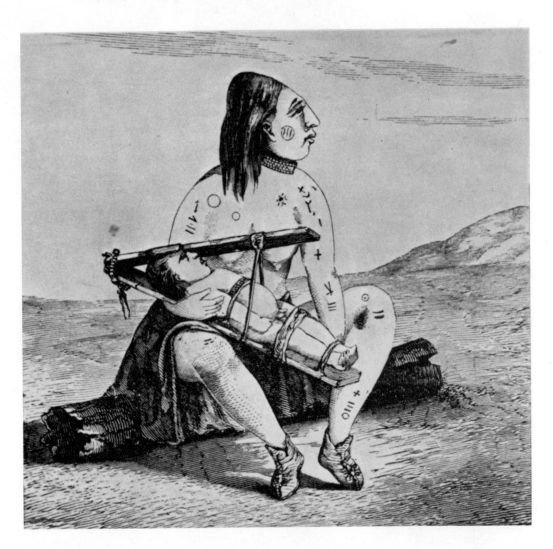

breathing, which alone would seem to justify their popularity. "Respiratory excitement," noted Havelock Ellis, "has always been a conspicuous part of the whole process of tumescence and detumescence, of the struggles of courtship and of its climax. . . . any restraint upon muscular and emotional activity generally, tends to heighten the state of sexual excitement."[96] For example, the tightening of one's belt to the limit of endurance induces fantasies of being strangled, one of the more extreme, not to say conclusive, stages of love-making.

Ever since the erotic life of the infant was brought to light, we have been seeking explanations for the causes of an adult's aberrations in his earliest years. Thus, masochistic inclinations have been traced to the baby's unsuccessful efforts to break the ties of his swaddling clothes. At any rate, such information was volunteered by patients with total recall.[97] Furthermore, restriction of body movement, be it the hampering of the limbs or the bundling of the trunk, was early recognized as an essential quality of ceremonial dress. Both intensify personal awareness. In turn the tension of muscles and nerves expresses itself in unnatural behavior. The classical example is the military style of machinelike motion. The

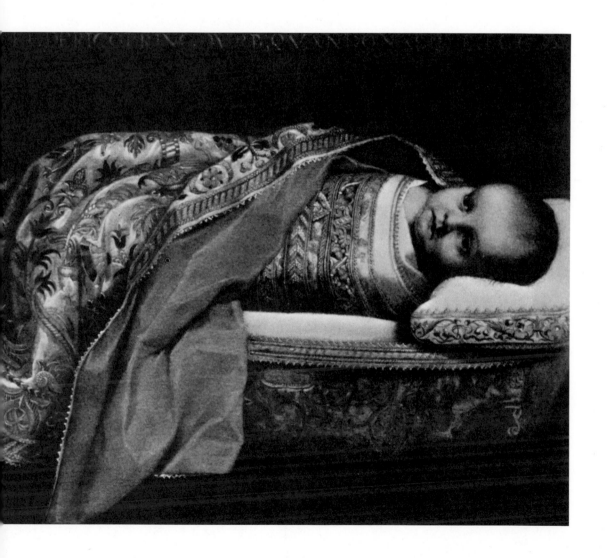

Portrait of Prince Federico di Urbino by Federico Barocci. 1605.

standing at "attention"—of which there is no parallel in the animal kingdom with its sharper faculties of *real* attention—the equally absurd marching in formations, the goose-stepping or the drill of chorus girls are but different aspects of the same phenomenon. As a rule, all these synchronized exertions call for uniform, often restricting, apparel.

The uniformed soldier has his counterpart in the harnessed and hobbleskirted woman. "We believe," wrote Hilaire Hiler, "that there may be such a thing as an anal-sadistic type of clothing which would be characterized by its tight fit, general stiffness and lack of

222

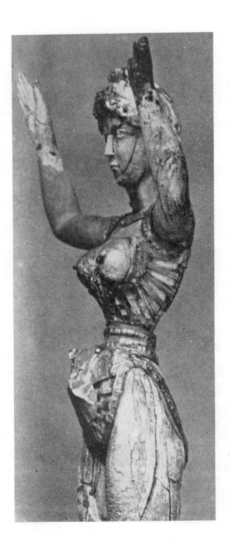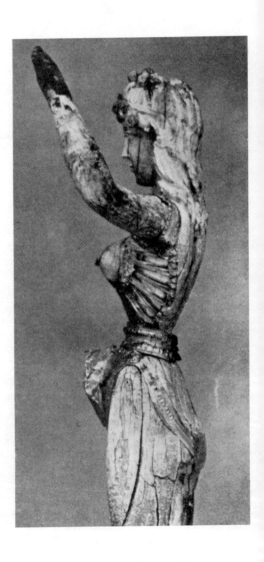

Minoan goddess, found in Crete. From Sir Arthur Evans, The Palace of Minos at Knossos.

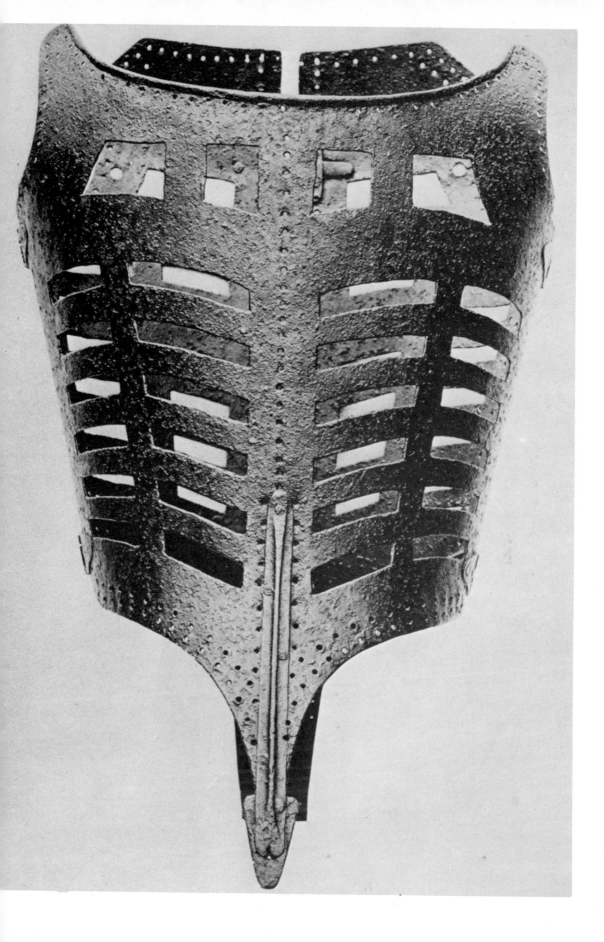

comfort. . . . for a number of years, women masochists, particularly, subjected themselves to the tortures of the now happily extinct corset as they still do to extremely high-heeled shoes."[98] Parenthetically, the corset is not gone forever; it survives in a kind of chrysalis from which it will emerge in its perfect cruelty at any moment propitious for its resurrection.

The discomfort experienced from wearing clothes varies considerably. The rib-cracking, toe-twisting paraphernalia that Western man used at various times to tenderize woman—much the way he cures meat to make it more savory—are largely unknown in the Orient, with two notable exceptions: Chinese foot binding, and the authentic kimono, the Japanese woman's straight jacket. The first will soon be but a memory; in a few years the last crippled woman will have disappeared, and with her one of the most perverse foot fashions ever invented. Only from poems and pictures shall we be able to reconstruct visions of fluttering females, balancing on their big toes, a sight as much relished by the Chinese of old as by our balletomanes. Today, Chinese men do without this national specialty and apparently have no difficulty making love to women with repulsively normal feet.

Japanese men, on the other hand, are more than reluctant to see the kimono go. Not that there is any danger at the moment that it might lose its popularity; after all, in its present form it is already one hundred years old, and there still seems enough life in it for a few more centuries to come. Its transformation from a pleasantly loose garment into a tight cocoon is due to the obi. Once a narrow ribbon for tying the outermost wrapper of the multi-layered garment, it deteriorated into a stiff sash as unwielding as a barrel hoop and many times as wide. Under its pressure the breasts are squashed and pushed down, the skin becomes discolored, sometimes making a woman's abdomen look as if it were permanently afflicted with Saint Anthony's fire. Yet the obi is but the finishing touch to the kimono, the genuine article, that is, not what *we* call a kimono. For a disciplinarian costume it looks deceptively innocent, not hinting at the intricate system of ties it harbors. On probing it, one discovers a curious rigging of cords and undergarments, drawn taut around the body, that immobilize the torso and glue the knees together. Only the lower part of the legs is allowed some amplitude —about twenty degrees—for walking. These restrictions account for a kimonoed woman's peculiar gait, a sort of half-step in which the toes are directed inward and the feet describe half-circular, scythelike movements. The point is that this kimono-conditioned walk becomes second nature to women. They assume it even when wearing Western clothes and shoes. Indeed, they are incapable of walking any other way.

Could it be that a natural walk is sexually unattractive? Once more a digression is in order.

At the age of about one, when a child develops from a quadruped into a biped, he gets up from all fours and learns to use his hind legs. As his confidence in them increases, he is tempted to run and jump and, if he happens to live in a non-urban environment, he may want to explore another dimension and climb trees. In the course of growing up, this childish urge to romp subsides, and by the time he approaches adulthood, he has formed a low opinion of walking. By then, walking, to his mind, is but one degree removed from his earlier experience of crawling on the floor.

There are, of course, exceptions. An abnormally energetic person may feel a call to devote the better part of his life to jumping high and far; more precisely, to jumping higher and farther than anybody else, or simply to running fast, not because there is any real need to negotiate obstacles in or out of doors, or to outdistance the other man in the street, but because a number of people are willing to pay for the privilege of watching others exert themselves. He may be considered a freak; he will find admirers but few imitators. By philistine standards, inertia ranks supreme; immobility confers dignity upon the meanest of men whereas walking beyond the barest necessity marks him a social misfit. Still, walking may not fall into oblivion altogether if only because it serves other functions as well. Although among so-called civilized nations the legs are being less and less employed for locomotion, the walk, particularly a stylish walk, conditioned by the harness of clothes and shoes, plays a singular rôle in man's love antics and thus in the propagation of mankind.

Darwin, the Spock of the species, was not above describing what

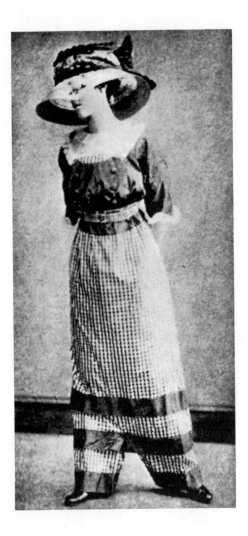

In 1911 fashionable women turned into mechanical toys with movements somewhat between a waddle and a sack race. From Vogue *magazine.*

he referred to as the "incredibly odd attitudes" and "extremely ludicrous parades" of courting birds, yet he does not mention the equally odd and ludicrous aspects of the human walk. To be sure, strutting males are mostly confined to the animal kingdom. The shambling gait of modern man—his legs encased, his arches preserved—hardly turns a woman's head. But then his walk is not meant to excite her; it is woman's business to do the prancing. If she is very good at it, her gait becomes her main attraction—so much so that it is diagnosed as a measure of sexual allure. For, as we shall see, a woman's attractiveness is determined less by the degree to which she reveals her body than by the way she walks.

A woman's natural gait—performed without interference from any kind of foot-gear—can still be observed in some out-of-the-way places of Asia and Africa. Watching a barefoot woman walk, one is surprised at how much her movements differ from those of a barefoot man. Even before she reaches full bloom, her carriage—the word is meant to include both framework and posture—betrays her sex. Buttocks and hips become conspicuous in walking, and sometimes are further emphasized by decorations. The Papuans, for

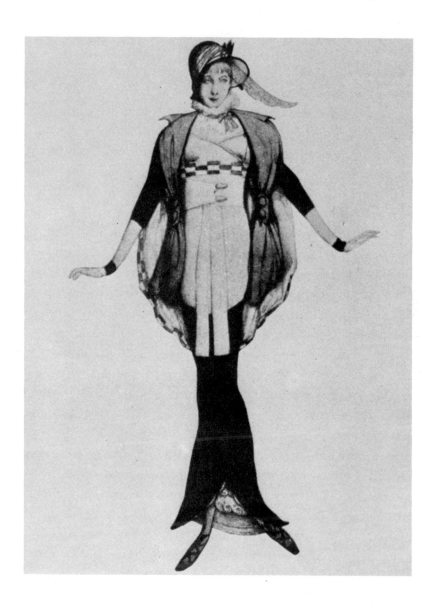

Although the handcuffs are only vestigial, the restriction of the hobbleskirt is very real. Drawing by Leon Bakst, 1912.

instance, have a high regard for the vibrating buttocks of their women who early learn to cultivate a provocative walk. At the age of seven or eight, a girl is taught the finer points of *vibrato*, an exercise of great delicacy, "and the Papuan maiden walks thus whenever she is in the presence of men, subsiding into a simpler gait when no men are present."

A woman's movements are no less alluring when she is fully clothed. Tertullian, the earliest of ancient church writers, complained in his treatise *De Pudicitia* that most women either from simple ignorance or from dissimulation, have the hardihood so to walk as if modesty consisted only in the integrity of the flesh. Yet it would seem that throughout classical antiquity, woman, whether housewife or goddess, got along without a coquettish walk. The stride of long-skirted, flat-sandaled women, recorded with camera-like precision on thousands of vases, was apparently devoid of artifice. The art of walking *seductively*—by curbing the freedom of the body's movements—was invented and perfected in the Orient.

The origin of restricting a woman's walk is lost in the tenebrous past. A hobbled horse or tethered goat at pasture may have suggested to a herdsman similarly to secure the women who were part of his goods and chattels. Thus, awkward footgear or heavy foot ornaments reduced them to a permanent state of real or mock captivity and, after a rustic honeymoon, a bride settled down in her role as domestic animal and slave. No doubt, she either accepted, or feigned, helplessness in order to please her man. Moreover, by suffering his caprices, she was able to turn the tables on him, and make *him* her slave.

In time her fetters became elaborate and precious, though no less effective and, like so many inconvenient acquisitions, ended up as status symbols. She probably flaunted her bonds as proudly as modern woman shows off her engagement ring. Man, for his part, became so absorbed in the subtleties of taming woman that he lost all interest in her clothes. Increasingly concerned with hiding her charms from his fellow men, he would see to it that she looked *un*attractive when leaving the house. Still, female ingenuity was able not only to cope with this further humiliation but to turn it into an added decoy:

Ancient Jewish female dress, one of apparel's dreariest types, is charitably omitted from costume histories, and with good reason. Out of doors, an honest woman resembled nothing so much as a shapeless bundle. And yet a man passing her in the street might have been shaken to the bones. Even with his eyes closed—indeed, a blind man could not help falling under her spell, which was transmitted, *mirabile dictu*, acoustically. What he heard was the sound of the jingle bells she carried under her skirts. Like the sleighbells on horses, they, too, were part of her harness. Stepping chains, Palestine's contribution to erotic accessories, joined the ankles together in a way that, according to the *Encyclopaedia Biblica*, "obliged the wearer to take short and tripping steps."[99] Concealed by long garments, the unconventional jewelry betrayed its presence

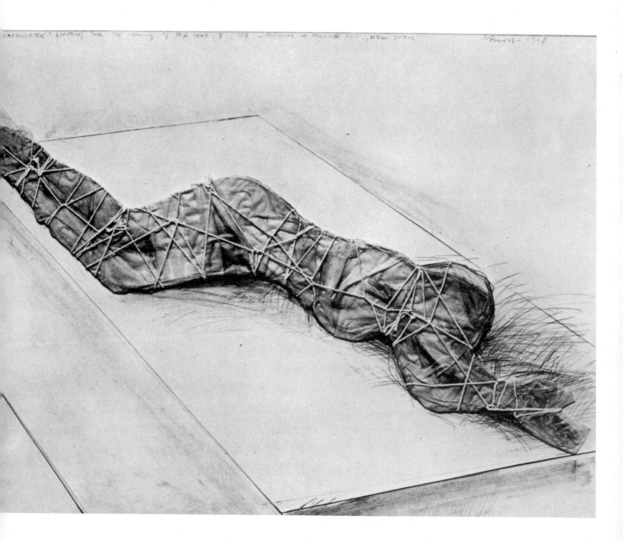

"Femme Empaquetée," (project) by Christo, 1968.

only by its tinkling and a woman's mincing walk. How admirable man's inventiveness, and woman's sense of humor, to make fun of a tyrannical scheme by setting the hobbled gait to musical accompaniment!

So deeply did this get-up affect the menfolk that it roused Isaiah to one of his inspired outbursts. A seer by profession, he felt duty bound to make his famous and, as it turned out, accurate forecast on the decline of women's finery: "The Lord will take away the beauty of their anklets, and the cauls, and the crescents; the pendants, and the bracelets, and the mufflers; the headtires, and the ankle chains."[100] Scholarly dissertations have been written on the elegant fetters and the intense sensations they cause. Condemned by moralists and moralizers, their popularity was assured by the ease with which they could be incorporated into the code of respectability.

Some African fashions convincingly prove that the egotism of the primitive is in no way inferior to that of civilized man. As one anthropologist noted, "the wives of some of the wealthy are often laden with iron to such a degree that, without exaggeration, I have seen several carrying about them close upon half a hundred-weight [50 lbs] of these savage ornaments."[101] (With Africans, iron is, or was, rare, and more precious than silver.) In Behar, Hindostan, the women wear brass rings on their legs. Each ring, an anthropological journal discloses, is nearly a foot wide and serrated around the edges. It can only be put on by a competent blacksmith, "who fits it on the legs of the women with his hammer while they writhe upon the ground in pain."[102] "The women of the Herero, similarly in ballast, "walk with a slow, dragging step which is considered aristocratic." The underprivileged among them who cannot afford the cyclopic jewelry have to be content with mimicking the awkward walk of the rich.

This compulsion to obstruct a woman's walk is far more widespread than one might think. In South-African Balonda, Livingstone notes, the favorite wife of a chief could be distinguished by "a profusion of iron rings on her ankles, to which were attached little pieces of sheet-iron, to enable her to make a tinkling as she walked in her mincing African style."[103] "The same thing," he adds with an unexpected flash of sarcasm, "is thought pretty by our own dragoons." Come to think of it, spurs, the alleged attributes of knighthood, correspond—at least acoustically—to the weighty status symbols of the primitive.

Exceptions may not always prove the rule yet there are tribesmen, and by no means only so-called savage ones, who derive satisfaction from practicing a bizarre walk, tugging at imaginary bonds or side-stepping invisible obstacles. According to Livingstone, Balonda men could be seen "with only a few ounces of ornament on their legs, strutting along as if they had double the number of pounds." There seems to be nothing particularly feminine about this mannerism; one has only to go to Japan to find its perfect equivalent among those paragons of virility, the actual or would-be descendants of samurai. Although the ancient warrior class was abolished generations ago, some Japanese men still walk astraddle, so to speak, planting their feet wide apart, simulating the gait of the samurai who was forever hampered by the two swords dangling from his waist belt. (The second sword symbolized a battle trophy, taken from a conquered enemy.) An extreme version of a choreographed walk is affected by the Japanese Emperor at ceremonies of state. His "jerky walk," the *New York Times* commented, "is one of style and not of chance or disability."[104]

An ingenious scheme for being in fashion without suffering its indignities is mentioned by Isabel Burton in her book on Syria and Palestine. Damascene women, she observed, had found a way to satisfy their vanity without sacrifice of comfort. At a wedding party, Mrs. Burton noticed that "the best women were dressed in a plain Cashmere robe of négligé shape, and wore no ornaments, but loaded all their riches on one or two of their slaves, as if to say, in schoolgirls' parlance: 'now girls, if you want to see my things, there they are . . .' "[105]

In our civilization the part played by foot chains and foot ornaments has been taken over in a desultory way by all sorts of bizarre footwear. Until a few hundred years ago, the wearing of stilts and stilted shoes was alien to the Western world; the custom was brought to Europe from the Orient. The port of entry was again Venice.

The seventeenth-century chronicler Thomas Coryat described the feminine footwear of the time as vividly as any modern fashion reporter: "There is one thing used of the Venetian women, and some others dwelling in the cities and towns subject to the Signiory of Venice, that is not to be observed (I think) amongst any other women in Christendom; which is so common in Venice, that no woman whatsoever goes without it, either in her house or abroad; a thing made of wood, and covered with leather of sundry colors, some with white, some red, some yellow. It is called a Chapiney, which they wear under their shoes. Many of them are curiosly painted; some also I have seen fairly gilt: so uncomely a thing (in my opinion) that it is pity this foolish custom is not clean banished and exterminated out of the city. There are many of these Chapineys of a great height, even a yard high, which makes many of their women that are very short, seem much taller than the tallest women

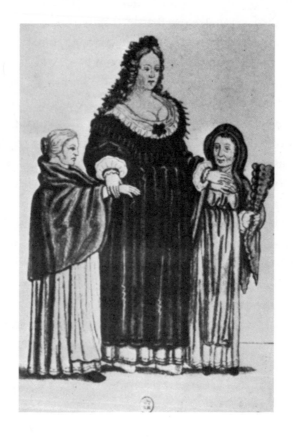

A variant of the Seeing Eye dog, these servants steer their towering mistress on a safe course through the streets of Venice. Water color by Gaignères, 1485.

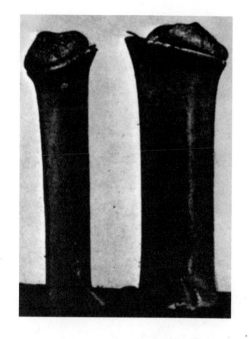

A pair of chopines, more than twenty inches high, instrument and symbol of woman's submission to man. Despite the Venetian authorities' efforts to outlaw the hazardous contraptions, they enjoyed popularity for centuries. Museo Civico, Venice.

we have in England. Also I have heard that this is observed amongst them, that by how much the nobler a woman is, by so much higher are her Chapineys. All their Gentlewomen, and most of their wives and widows that are of any wealth, are assisted and supported either by men or women when they walk abroad, to the end they may not fall. They are born up most commonly by the left arm, otherwise they might quickly take a fall. For I saw a woman fall a very dangerous fall, as she was going down the stairs of one of the little stony bridges with her high Chapineys alone by her self: but I did nothing pity her, because she wore such frivolous and (as I may truly term them) ridiculous instruments, which were the occasion of her fall."[106]

Chopines had been banned almost two hundred years before Coryat's time. In 1430, when they reached a height of more than twenty inches, the Venetian government prohibited their use. The fathers of the Republic, noticing their potential dangers, feared that pregnant women who stumbled on the rough pavement of the town, would give birth to *filios abortivos in perditione corporis et animae suae*.[107] Yet the chopine stayed on. It was instrumental in changing the proportion, posture and gait of a woman; in the light of costume history we may consider it of singular momentousness. Until then, men and women had been, literally, on equal footing. Allowing for differences in their steps and paces, their carriage had remained fairly natural. Now, with the elevating shoe of the East having gained a foothold on Europe, a woman's shoe would never again be mistaken for a man's except during that short period in the eighteenth century when also men wore high heels.

During the sixteenth and seventeenth centuries the wearing of stilted shoes became fashionable in other European countries. Women of short stature delighted in their use, all the more as long skirts hid the clumsy contraptions. Brantôme in his *Vie des Dames*

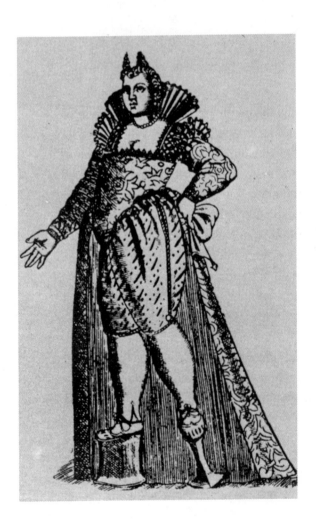

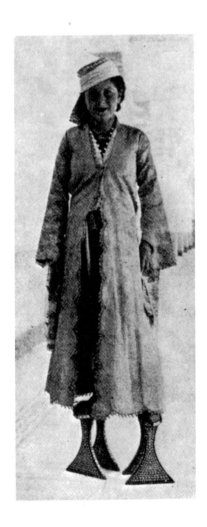

Left: A peep under the skirt of a Venetian courtesan reveals the artifice of her footwear.
From Pietro Bertelli's Diversarum Nationum Habitus.

Right: Syrian bride wearing nuptial pede
From Géographie, 1939.

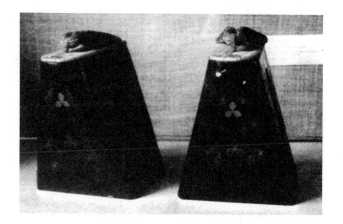

Far from stooping to anything as homely as "walking shoes," Japanese courtesans wore high clogs as a professional attribute.

Galantes mentions that Frenchwomen wore clogs as much as two feet high, and a visitor to the court of Madrid noted that even the queen of Spain, the wife of Philip V, walked on *chopins*. To do this she had to rely on the support of two helpers, like a Venetian courtesan.

The excessive height of these shoes—some look more like furniture than apparel—transformed women into strange creatures hovering high above the ground. Yet it was by no means their weird elongation alone that pleased the men. The continued attraction of the portable footstools was based on their instability; the sight of a woman walking precariously closely corresponded to man's image of feminine helplessness. The special appeal of this type of footwear can be inferred from the frequency with which it appeared in courting and marriage ceremonies. Syrian kubkabs—the onomatopoetic word for the clogs from which the Venetian chopines are descended—are made absurdly high for brides.

At the other end of Asia, in Kyoto's ancient red light district Shimabara (now exorcised of all evil to pacify the Puritan tourist), a reasonable facsimile of the Great Whore is led through the streets at an annual procession still held in our time. Her outfit includes sandals that are twelve inches high. For balance and support she depends on two female apprentices. She moves painfully slowly, as gingerly as if she were moving backward, "dragging the heavy wooden pedestals by her toes only—a grand spectacle of sex appeal."[108] These forms of castigation, or exhibitionism—the point of view depending on one's sex—have been somewhat mitigated by an increasing number of social taboos, but the intensity of male egotism has not lessened.

The sex appeal of an unnatural walk persists. It has been diagnosed by Havelock Ellis as "an almost abstract fascination in the idea of restraint, whether endured, inflicted, or merely witnessed or imagined; the feet become the chief focus of this fascination, and the basis on which foot-fetichism or shoe-fetichism tends to arise, because restraint of the feet produces a more marked effect than restraint of the hands."[109] The various foot ornaments and foot coverings of costume history could not have withstood the changes of taste had it not been for their elementary appeal to the senses, i.e. the "voluptuous emotions" they release in wearer and beholder. "Pain itself," maintained Ellis, "may under a great variety of special circumstances become an erotic symbol and afford the same relief as the emotions normally accompanying the sexual act."[110]

Garments for two

Has anybody ever heard of a garment for two? And I don't mean the kind of sports outfits for him and her that once were worn by tandem-riding cyclists, nor those mother-and-daughter dresses which are identical except for size; or, least of all, clothes for Siamese twins. What I have in mind is a single garment that accommodates two ordinary people, more precisely, adults of opposite sex. No such garment is made here or abroad, nor can it be found in museums. In fact, it is unknown to either museum curators, dress designers, or garment manufacturers. The garment in question simply never made its way into sewing manuals, costume books, or for that matter into *any* book that appeared during the past three and a half centuries.

A garment for two was first mentioned in the pages of *Indiae Orientalis,* a work of many volumes by several authors. *Indiae* was never translated into English. It was published in Latin in 1612, and deals largely with the Dutch admiral Pierre Willemsz Verhoeven's five-year-long exploits in the Moluccas, an island group in the Malay Archipelago, south of the Philippines. Verhoeven had orders to bolster Dutch rule in the islands by destroying all Portuguese settlements in them, a task he performed in a consummate manner. As might be expected, the book makes pleasant reading for the sanguinary only; it abounds with descriptions of massacres and incendiarism, acts that have long come to be associated with colonizing and proselytizing. Not until the ninth volume does the work strike a peaceful note. That part contains the memoires of one John Vercken, alias Jean Verck, a ship's officer of Verhoeven's fleet. Upon receiving his discharge, Verck decided to visit some of the archipel's larger islands and to indulge his bent for observing exotic surroundings. With fighting out of the way, and with enough time to do some exploring of his own, he began to record his impressions in punctilious detail. Of special interest are his notes on popular customs and costumes in the islands of Celebes, Java and Sumatra.

It was on Sumatra that he saw women wearing what struck him as an uncommon body covering. Reaching no farther than to the knees, it was open at the top and bottom but completely closed all around. What it lacked in length, it made up in width. In order to put it on, Verck explained, a woman slipped it over her head and fastened it under her arms. Although today we are inured to such artlessness, to Verck the dress seemed an extraordinarily clever invention. Not that he thought it particularly attractive. On the contrary, it reminded him, as he said, of a sack. However, conditioned as he was to seventeenth-century wasp waists, he could not help admiring its stark simplicity. At any rate, the dress was ingenuous enough to merit a second look, and Verck soon realized that there was more to it than meets the eye. To quote: "Virum admittere volentes, saccu istu sub brachiis colligatum soluunt, viroq; simul iniiciunt, satis occulte res suas peragere se posse sperantes, si vterq; in sacco haereant."[111] Which means, rendered freely, if a woman wants to admit a man, she unfastens her dress and pulls it over both, believing that they will be sufficiently concealed.

Although *Indiae* is heavily illustrated, the garment's peculiar collateral aspect is nowhere shown. Maybe this is just as well since nearly all the early travelers were poor at pictorial reporting. Few of them were good draftsmen, and the others, who combined a discriminating eye with a talent for drawing, had their hands full of more important things to do than to bother about the strange and picturesque. Moreover, none of the explorers seems to have thought of the obvious—to hire a professional artist. Apparently it never occurred to Columbus to ask Leonardo—a man notoriously fond of sketching—to come along on his voyage into the unknown. The habit of including a full-time draftsman on an expeditionary force developed only much later; most early travel reports were illustrated by stay-at-homes. Conscientious artists though they were, they depended entirely on accounts by word of mouth which frequently were confusing, contradictory, or highly exaggerated. Since imagination had to make up for the scarcity of evidence, it is not surprising that the old books contain many fanciful pictures—bucolic scenes where rhinoceros and unicorn graze side by side, improbable works of architecture, and even more improbable human creatures. Whatever the artist's talent for depicting the exotic and remote, when it came to rendering an unfamiliar costume—a feat that demands a lot more than proficiency in drawing—he was at a loss. But then, to correctly assess the dimension and "cut" of a garment from the way it looks on a person is quite difficult and often downright impossible, as many a fashion pirate has learned to his chagrin. To wit, the shape of a garment as basic as the Roman toga remained a puzzle for nearly two thousand years; despite the silent testimony of countless toga-clad statues, its true outline was not known until the nineteenth century. No wonder that Verck's description of the Sumatran dress was not supplemented by as much as a diagrammatic sketch.

The use of apparel as a matrimonial tent was by no means restricted to Sumatra; on Celebes Verck observed a full-length male variant of the same garment. The men, he wrote, have a nethergarment to cover their privy parts, but sometimes they also have a long, wide sack which they carry tucked around their waist. When worn, it reaches from head to foot. "However, they don't put it on," he explained, "until they want to be with a woman. Then they slip it over both of them, remaining concealed from peoples' eyes."

If Verck was astonished to see a garment double as a trysting place, he did not say so. Neither did he have words of censure for the outlandish spectacle, but then his century was more enlightened than ours. To people brought up on monosexual clothes, garments for two seem frivolous if not altogether indecent. Therefore it must come as a surprise to most of us to learn that such clothes play a prominent part in the rites of a number of communities. As ceremonial garments they have a long tradition in the East Indies where they have been invested with something like sacramental qualities. "Union in marriage and other rites," one reads in an ethnological essay, "is commonly effected by enveloping the pair *in one robe.*"[112] (Italics added.) A similar sleight-of-hand has been met with in the Malay Peninsula. There, marriages are contracted mostly at harvest time—a thanksgiving observance which the Encyclopaedia Britannica archly calls "a marriage carnival." According to native etiquette, on the wedding day the groom betakes himself to the bride's house. The ceremony that follows is unlike anything we know. The pair is placed together and covered with a cotton fabric. After several hours, their twosomeness comes to a grinding halt. The cover is removed "and they are man and wife."[113]

At a glance there is something very engaging about this hide-and-seize. It may not be distinguished for refinement, yet it is shot through with the innocent sensuality one finds in ancient tales. "In South Celebes," writes an ethnologist, "the ceremony of Ridjala Sampù consists in enveloping [the bridal pair] in one sarong, which the priest casts over them like a net."[114] No picture accompanies the text, but at least the garment is identified as a sarong—a loose skirt, made of a long strip of cloth, wrapped around the body and held in place by tucking or rolling at the waist. It is worn chiefly by the men and women of the Malay archipelago and the Pacific islands. Marsden, in his *History of Sumatra,* says that it is "not unlike a Scott's highlander plaid in appearance, being a piece of party colored cloth about six or eight feet long, and three or four wide, sewed together at the ends; forming a wide sack without bottom. This is sometimes gathered up, and flung over the shoulder like a sash, or else folded and tucked about the waist and hips."[115] From the available sources it appears that on Sumatra and the neighboring islands of Borneo and Nias, the uniting of the bridal pair in a single garment is, or was, part and parcel of the wedding ceremony.[116] But what is one to make of the fact that the same custom obtains on Madagascar, five thousand miles distant from Celebes?[117] Surely, the points of similarity bespeak a widespread tradition of garments for two, both sacramental and bawdy.

In this cozy world of symbols, the stark reality of Verck's garment —as I shall call it for convenience's sake—reappears in, of all places, North America. American aborigines seem to have discovered its merits independently from the rest of the world. This domestic version of a blind for casual dallying is described in Dodge's *Our Wild Indians,* a book written shortly before the turn of the century. Although the garment in question is not quite the tubular type that promises privacy in the round, it is the nearest approximation, a wraparound. Since we are here on home ground, far from the Banda Sea, a full quotation seems in order: "There is a vast amount of love-making in an Indian camp," wrote Colonel R. I. Dodge, "for aside from that common and natural to unmarried youths of both sexes, the custom of most Plains tribes makes every man a possible suitor for the hand of every woman, though either or both may be already married." The prospective lover, wrapped in a Buffalo robe or a wide cotton cloak, stalks his prey by night and, as soon as she slips out of her lodge, pounces upon her. At first they stand facing each other, each wrapped in his own garment. "If the affair progresses favorably, they still remain standing, but find one blanket or robe sufficient for both." "Couples so engaged," adds the author reassuringly, "are never disturbed."[118]

A vanished world to be sure, yet so elementary is the appeal of an open-air outfit which guarantees some measure of privacy that, had it never existed, it would need to be invented. As happens so often, imagination is on the side of the novelist rather than on that of the novelty monger. To wit, in a pastoral passage of *For Whom the Bell Tolls,* Hemingway introduced a garment for two, albeit a horizontal one, the *Beischlafsack,* which serves Robert Jordan as his roost in the Spanish woods. He literally bags his stray Maria by asking her to share his warmth. *"Get in," he said softly, ". . . Just slip in. There is much room. Do you want me to help you?" "No," she said and then was in the robe.* Hemingway calls it a sleeping robe, a singular genteelism in a book which teems with racy language.

Variations of actual or symbolic coupling by means of apparel occur among many peoples who kept their rituals intact. A highly stylized union by sartorial merger takes place in a number of wedding ceremonies where bride and groom are tied together. The Hindus call this the Brahman knot. An analogous method of pairing is practiced on the American continent; the Tarahumare of Mexico cover the bridal couple with blankets and tie their hands together. For a more capricious example, in the Old China the hair of the bridegroom was fastened to that of the bride. Intimacy of this kind is further intensified by serving the couple their wedding dinner on a single plate. This is a parallel to making love in Verck's garment. Apart from the symbolic connotations of eating—in the Scriptures "eating" is often a rank euphemism for coitus—conviviality is not everybody's dish; some people consider the physical act of food ingestion a most private affair. To them, eating in company is nothing short of indecent. This phobia is not limited to individuals; a number of tribes cannot bring themselves to eat in public although they feel no shame when going naked. To conceal the act of eating is imperative to them while to cover the body is not.

To judge from stray references, vestiges of Verck's garment in the form of clothes, blankets or just plain pieces of fabric are used at wedding ceremonies in a number of countries. They are held above the couple's heads as a magic umbrella against the fallout of divine wrath. Such need for protection against the dangers from above was early turned to good account in ancient Egypt, where a bride walked under a canopy. Scarcely less arresting, though admittedly more ambiguous instances of this usage can be found in Europe thousands of years later. Symbolic shelter is admirably illustrated in a Renaissance painting (artist unknown) of a wedding procession where an outdoor canopy for the bride and her party forms a continuous cover all the way from the parental house to the church. A simpler and thriftier solution called for a Jewish bride to ride in a covered litter. The wedding ceremony proper made up for what the procession lacked. It took place under a tent, a square of satin or silk, stretched across the top of four poles from which developed the *chuppah*, or *qubbah*, the canopy still used in orthodox weddings. The non-denominational version of the chuppah and ultimate reduction of the marital cover, stylized out of recognition, is the less than ascetic *ciel de lit,* or *Betthimmel,* the canopy of the fourposter bed.

Although Americans never caught up with the lore of either East or West India, in recent years novel garments were launched by people who had togetherness uppermost in mind. Among these far-out creations was a "sweater for two," put on the market by a Californian knitwear manufacturer. A plaything for the young, it **243** falls short, however, of being a portable tunnel of love. Even though its name has a distinctly copulative ring, it possesses none of the amenities of Verck's garment. As can be seen from the photograph, the sweater joins a couple, much like Siamese twins, at their sides.

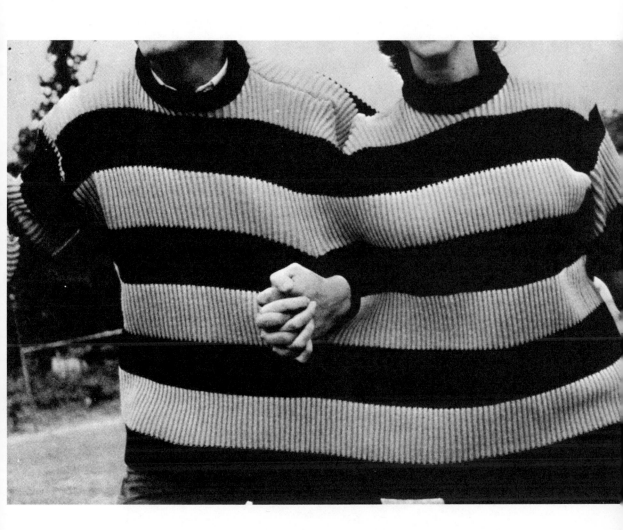

Sweater for two. 1963. (Courtesy, Trend Fashions)

Allowing as it does for some left-handed caresses under cover, essentially it holds the two at bay. An embrace would split it wide open.

Another timid venture into pluralistic apparel is a sleeping bag for two pairs of feet that made its debut in this country a few years ago. The idea behind it would seem excellent in more than one respect. Cold feet—in the actual and figurative sense—are common enough; more importantly, the foot has always been considered a focus of sexual attraction. At least this is true for a number of European countries where touching the coveted person's feet is an ancient form of courting. Traditionally practiced at table as a sort of counterpoint to dinner conversation, it serves as a secret feeler be-

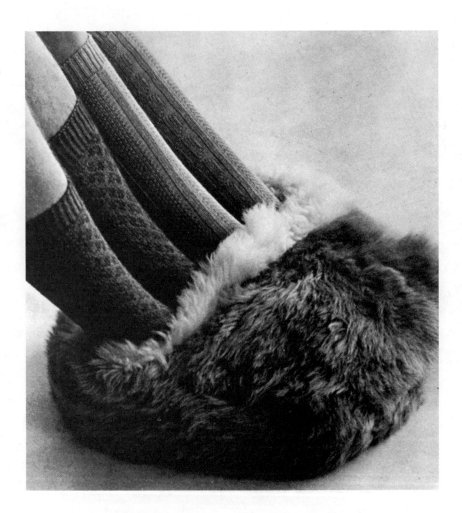

Footwarmer. 1966. (Courtesy, Josephine Creel. Iberian Imports)

tween prospective lovers, a pedal variant of holding hands. The custom, which originated among peasants who either go barefoot most of the time or wear slipperlike wooden clogs, has no application hereabouts since epidermal contact is essential. According to Wildhagen's English-German Dictionary, *füsseln* means "to foot it; to make love with one's feet under the table." It seems that as a transmitter of emotions the foot is vastly superior to the hand; "The hand," noted the American psychologist G. Stanley Hall, "does not possess the mystery which envelops the foot."[119]

In theory, then, a furry playpen for two pairs of feet is made to order for stimulating jaded appetites; it would seem to hold the promise of unthought-of excursions into voluptuousness. Alas, the novelty shown here misses out on this point for it is clearly designed to *segregate* the feet. It represents little more than a belated footnote on courting, New England style, the quaint rite of bundling. As a further precaution, the legs of the would-be lovers are encased—at least in the accompanying picture—in heavy no-nonsense stockings, an accessory that cannot but wreck the charms of the flesh. The quadruped footwear is probably not even intended to arouse passionate feelings but merely to kindle the pale fire of marital bliss and to keep going in unison a sluggish blood circulation.

Clothes and the artist

For more than 40,000 years, a stretch of time that is hard to grasp, fullblooded artists delighted in portraying the human form. They sculpted and painted it in praise of man and, for want of a better model, in praise of God as well. They went about their work with awe rather than fear; on their aesthetic scale, supernatural beings took precedence over mortal ones perhaps because they presented a greater challenge to their imagination. Unfortunately, this challenge was not met; it is a sad comment on the artists of all times that they fell short of inventing a divine icon that was *not* earthbound. What prevented them from finding full scope for their skill was the uncommon difficulty of translating the deity into a comprehensible image. Try as they might to sustain a high pitch of creativity, the materialization on canvas or in stone of a being superior to man was beyond their powers. For one thing, their own visions and dreams did not disclose to them the sort of elements from which to construct a sublime figure; for another, those saints and near-saints who were privileged to consort with creatures from another world, failed to come up with inspiring descriptions of their visitors' likeness.

God's image does not exist in concrete form. In the religious sense He is invisible and unknowable, even though—in the Old Testament for instance—He manifested Himself as fire, smoke or a cloud, guises borrowed from Greek mythology. (Moses managed to see the Lord's back but not His face.) Besides, the Bible does mention God walking through the Garden of Eden, and closing the door of the Ark, and in apocryphal literature He is "roaring like a lion" and "weeping over the destruction of the Temple." Nowhere, however, is anything specific said about His looks. The artist, wrestling with the intractable truths of the Scriptures, is forever left to his own devices.

In order then to make God's presence truly felt; to give shape and color to the ineffable, the artist had to turn to anthropomorphism, the attribution of human form and human feelings to the deity. Essentially a blasphemous undertaking, it conferred upon man the honor of serving as a stand-in for the supreme being. Once, however, the artist had committed himself to this *quid pro quo,* he never succeeded in breaking away from the human shape. Even the most devout among them felt no qualms to contrive God in their own image, thus reversing the act of Creation.

As it happens when the artist meets defeat in dealing with the corporeal substance, whether godly or human, he has recourse to abstraction. The Church makes use of the same stratagem by enclosing the Host in the monstrance, the vessel exhibited at mass or carried in procession to be adored by the faithful. Usually, it is lavishly ornamented, often encrusted with jewels and, more significantly, wreathed with a golden gloriole. Gold, perhaps on account of its stability and resplendent luster, was early connected with holiness; in Christian iconography, a surfeit of gold leaf lights up the sky with perpetual fireworks. However, excessive beatitude stifles the most ardent talent. The artist, at a loss as to how to infuse God's image with otherworldliness, expended himself on the abstract heavenly background. Glories, aureoles, and darting rays, a galaxy of brilliances, almost obscure the holy pictures.

In contrast to its flashy frame, the deity breathes unmitigated humility. From the thirteenth century on, the effigy of God the Father has been an unsmiling old man, and nobody has improved on it ever since. Whatever its merits, it reduces the almighty to the mighty, the unknowable to the familiar. The only way to distinguish Him from a prophet is to show Him suspended in mid-air. Levitation, a phenomenon rarely observed on earth but well known to every astronaut, is His divine prerogative.

During the time when the Church nearly came to monopolizing art, the artist labored hard to bring the invisible universe within the believer's reach. He did his best work when literacy still ranked among life's luxuries and God's message was mainly transmitted by word of mouth. The more learned and fastidious the artist, the more difficult was his task. In his eagerness to reconcile theology with art he had to face problems of dress that would have discouraged a philosopher, let alone a tailor. The only way out of his dilemma was to fall back on the time-honored model of sartorial respectability—flowing Greek robes, usually starched in the Byzantine fashion.

Christian faith does not permit Him to shine in the nudity of the ancient gods. It prefers to clothe the divine form, thus making it share Adam's incompleteness. One might say that a good deal of the confusion that besets our ideas of modesty and dress can be traced to generations of artists who tried to solve the insolvable; who for want of a better idea subjected Him to their own questionable ethics by covering Him with ordinary garments. Clothes, the sticking plaster for original sin, thus came back to Him full circle.

Among the Hebrews where God's image was taboo, He was spared such masquerading. Unfortunately, this was the people's loss since the figurative arts never had a chance to take root in their life. In Protestant countries ecclesiastic arts fared little better. As late as in the nineteenth century, they had not recovered from Puritanism's blight. Ruskin bemoaned the "pre-eminent *dullness* [his italics] which characterizes what Protestants call sacred art; a dullness not merely baneful in making religion distasteful to the young, but sickening all vital belief of religion in the old."[120] Nothing much has changed in this respect.

The Church that sanctioned anthropomorphism balked at zoomorphism not without, however, allowing for a few exceptions. Christ sometime becomes a lamb or a fish; the Holy Ghost appears as a dove. Doubtless, such small deviations brought cheer to the artist who envied his colleagues of ancient times their greater freedom. To the painter of madonnas and saints the heathen gods with heads of lion, jackal, ape and hawk, that proliferated in Mesopotamia's sunny civilizations, must have seemed truly out of this world compared to his own humdrum creations. Contrary to what one might expect, a saint is not degraded by being equipped with an animal's head; the evangelists Mark, Luke, and John attain barbarous grandeur when represented as lion, bull, and eagle, respectively. Indeed, the question arises whether a judicious sprinkling of such paganisms might not have helped to strengthen people's

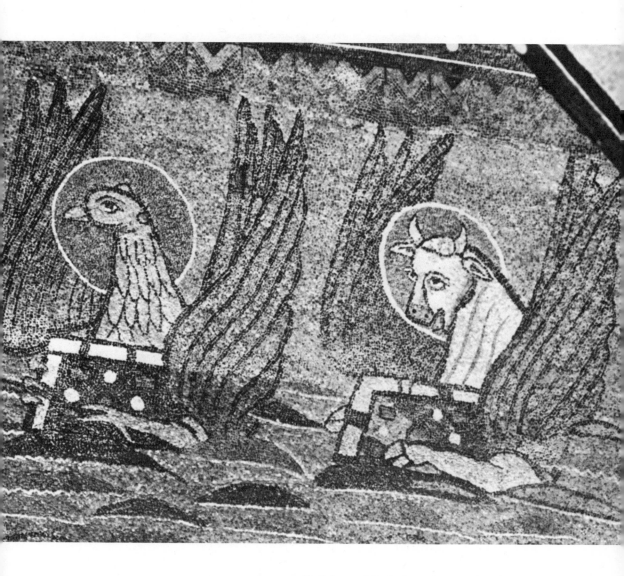

*St. John and St. Luke, metamorphosed and haloed.
Ninth-century mosaic. Sta. Prassede, Rome.*

faith in God. Would a deity with three faces not have impressed popular imagination as favorably as it did in other cultures? Sure enough, some artists who thought that their talents ought not to be confined by doctrine took a hint from double-faced Janus and transmuted the trinity of God the Father, the Son, and the Holy Ghost into a triple-faced image. But the clergy did not go along with them; they probably felt that such literal rendering of a hoary theological paradox—the archetype of the triadic divinity antedates Christianity by many centuries—might open a Pandora's paint box and lead back to idolatory.

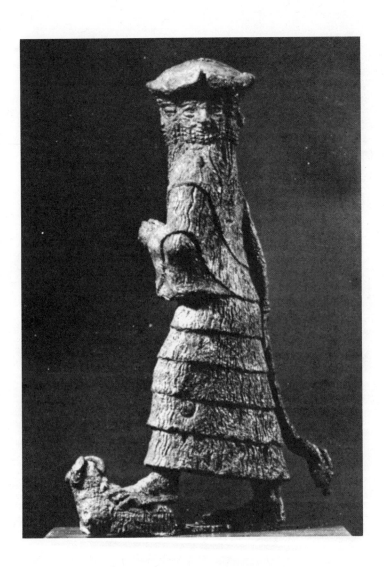

Bronze statuette of a four-faced god. Nineteenth century B.C. *Iraq; Ishchali.*
(Courtesy, Oriental Institute, University of Chicago)

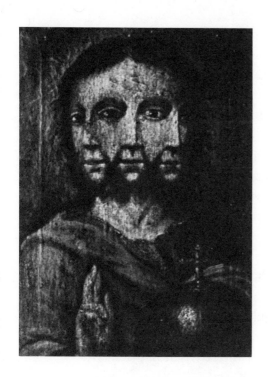

Idols with multiple faces occur in religious art of nearly every persuasion. Three-faced Christian Trinity. (Courtesy, Tiroler Volkskundemuseum, Innsbruck)

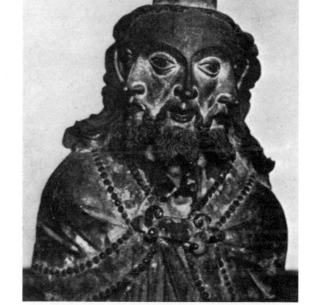

Medieval and Renaissance representations of three-faced Trinities were still venerated in the nineteenth century. Wood sculpture. Austrian, c. 1520. (Courtesy, Volkskundemuseum, Vienna)

When tackling angels, the next-holy subject, artists striving for visible holiness may often have found that there, too, the odds were against them. Angels are a brittle breed. They are by godly design unemotional and superlatively bland. Moreover, unlike saints and martyrs, they have no personal history; they had no share in Creation where they merely played the part of admiring onlookers. Yet their passivity notwithstanding, they are infinitely more portrayable than God Himself. They have always constituted an indispensable ingredient of heaven; without them heaven simply would be sky.

The earliest representations of Christian angels were found in catacombs. All of them are male—young men dressed in a tunic or pallium. They have neither wings nor halo. Not until the sixth century did angels begin to conform to the latter-day cliché of winged women with flowing hair and nondescript garments. Although wingless angels may be acceptable to theologians, they cut no ice with the pious. Hence the Church took a leaf out of the pagans' book and appropriated the wings of the Assyrian-Babylonian guardian angel, a hybrid, half woman, half bird.

According to Christian doctrine, the word angel stands for a great variety of heavenly creatures, winged and wingless, ranging from humble messengers to fierce destroyers (see Sodom, Gen. 19, and the Assyrian Army, II Kings 19:35). The four archangels, models of elegance, occupy the top of the hierarchy without, however, attaining the popularity of a cherubim or a seraphim, two species that make the greatest demands on the artist's creative faculties. Idiomatically, the cherub is but a chubby child—the baptized cupid—usually shown as a playmate of the Christ child. In biblical terms though, the word refers to a formidable flying machine powered by mystic energy, a four-faced, four-winged creature with whirling wheels. (Sculptors prefer to stay away from them.) According to Enoch (18:5), cherubim serve as vehicles that move along their own pathways; viz., the Lord flies through the heavens "mounted on a cherubim" (II Sam. 22:11, Ps. 18:11). Jewish religion denies the cherubim their angelhood; cherubim, says a Jewish encyclopaedia, were impersonal, mechanical beings.

More powerful than a cherubim is the seraphim—literally "the flaming one." An angel with three pairs of wings, he uses only one

The portraiture of a seraphim, the most advanced model of an angel, poses near-unsolvable problem none is ever shown in flight. The twelfth-century mosaic in the cathedral of Monreale presents a seraphim with his landing gear down, balancing three apostles on his shoulders. The hint of a skirt only adds to the mystery of his clothes' cut. As a rule he is naked.

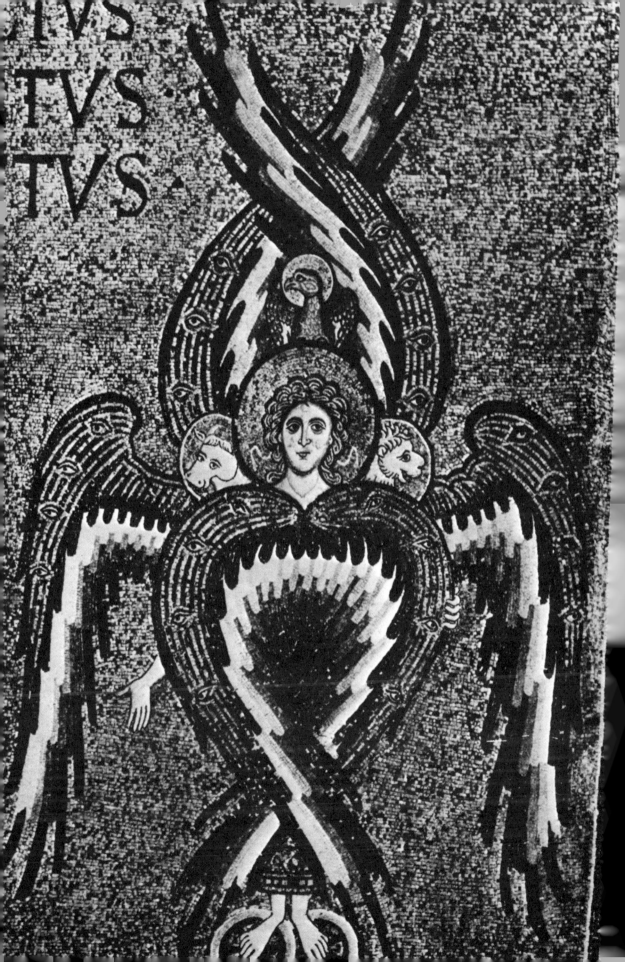

pair in flight and with the other two covers his loins and face. A triple bird, he interests us sartorially rather than aeronautically; he is all feathers and does not wear a stitch. His complicated structure, which would seem to make it impossible for him to get into clothes, exempts him from modesty's requirements.

The Fathers of the Church took a more sober view of angels by endowing them with "ethereal" bodies—the good ones bathing in radiant splendor, the bad ones (the devils) wrapped in "dark fuliginous obscurity." These specifications were of no help to artists. For one thing, piety kept them from guessing at an angel's anatomy. For another, they never could agree among themselves on where to put his wings. Hence instead of growing laterally, as they do on most animals, angels' wings sprout in the most unlikely places. Either they are attached to the shoulder blades or, more rarely, to hips and temples. As a result of their heavy plumage, they often look cumbersome. Fallen angels, on the other hand, are of more advanced design; they come equipped with bat wings that fold like an umbrella.

Whatever the arguments for or against their holiness, angels are Christianity's largest concession to people's need for some variety in the heavenly pageant. To judge from Christian iconography, they bore the brunt of the artist's adoration; in the celestial realm he felt free to indulge his infatuation with the birdwomen. Unlike man's image, theirs left a comfortable margin for inventiveness. Not that he was altogether spared some criticism. One militant angelologist lashed out at the absurdity of investing angels with a "puerile childishness of appearance," which was at variance with the divine design—"baby faces between a pair of bird's wings, destitute of bodies; slender girls with long and flowing ringlets, and the appendages of pinions well feathered with silvery plumes, so palpably destitute of the terrible grandeur and ethereal glory with which God had invested those illustrious and beautiful ambassadors of his rainbow throne and imperial sovereignty."[121] Today's children, familiar as they are with modern flying techniques, may see in an angel's wings little more than an ornament, about as supernatural as Santa's beard.

Winged creatures have always been associated with the power of

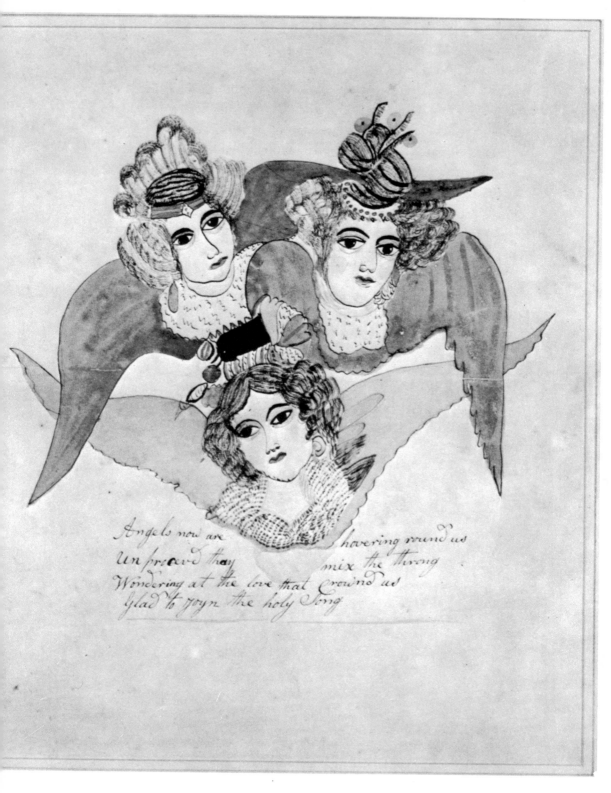

"Three Angel heads," by Mary Ann Willson, c. 1830.
(Courtesy, Museum of Fine Arts, Boston)

positive thought. The most intellectual of winged sphinxes, that of Thebes, was so intent on her calling that she literally devoured those who failed to answer her riddles. A less aggressive, air-born hybrid is Pegasus, half horse, half angel, the symbol of Mobil oil and poetry. Quite apart from winged bulls, winged lions and winged snakes, wings are standard equipment of most insects and birds who are but miniature editions of the fabulous flying monsters of the past, the dragons that gave battle to St. George and St. Michael. Only a modest mammalian aerial circus survives—flying squirrels, lemurs, fish and snakes. To man, however, wings proper are denied.

The human body—which does contain a few non-essential parts like the caecum—might have been improved no end by the addition of one or several pairs of wings. While the cut of clothes would thus have been further complicated, the gift of organic flight might have had its compensations. One of the few men who tried to correct this deficiency was the Greek sculptor-architect Daedalus. Having incurred the displeasure of his patron and client Minos, he

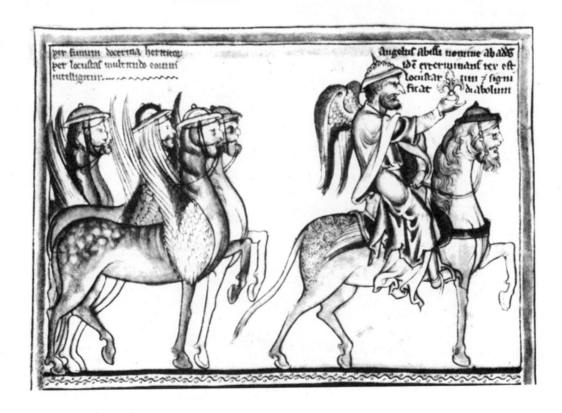

"Scenes from the Apocalypse." Manuscript, about 1240–60.
(Courtesy, The Trustees of the Pierpont Morgan Library)

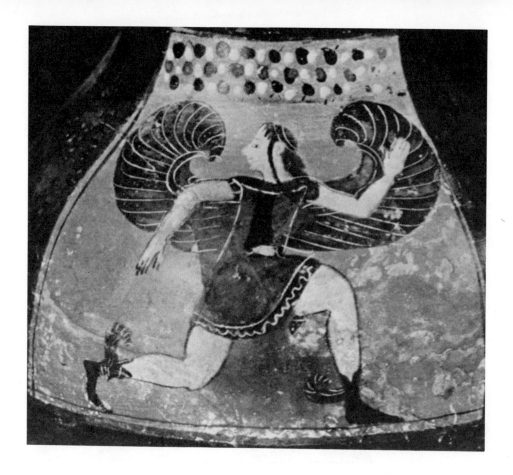

Bird women once were as ubiquitous as the common housefly. In the guise of nymphs, fairies, erotes, harpies, geni, etc., they wrought havoc among mortal men. Usually their love was lethal. Above: The vase painting, c. 580 B.C., shows a winged Nike, goddess of victory.

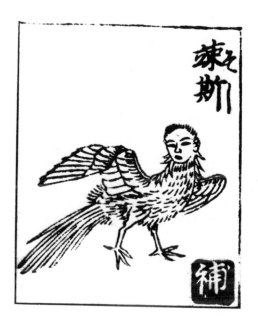

The human-faced bird (left) comes from a Japanese encyclopedia.

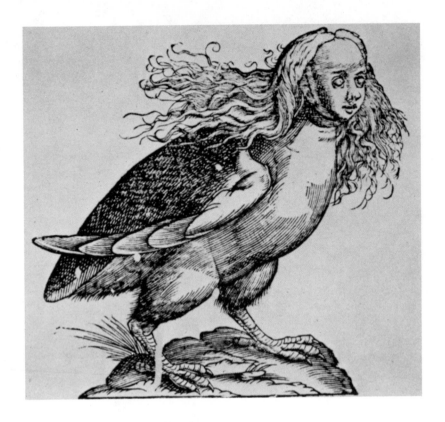

fashioned—probably with Psyche's airworthiness in mind—two pairs of wings, one for himself and one for his son Icarus, and escaped by air. As every schoolchild knows, disaster overtook them in midflight. *Already was Samos on their left (Naxos and Paros had been passed); on their right was Lebynthos and Calymne shady with forests, and Astypalaea girt with fish-haunted seas; when the boy, too bold in his youthful daring, deserted his sire and winged his way too high.*[122] The son crashed but the father successfully completed the five-hundred-mile flight from Crete to Sicily, and later, on the mainland (at Cumae) built a temple to Apollo as a token of thanks. Aware as he was of the historical importance of his feat, he bequeathed his wings to the holy place, thus adding a touch of the Smithsonian to it.

Only reluctantly did men abandon the idea of flying by the strength of their muscles. In a way though, they never relinquished it altogether; their hope simply went underground where it persists

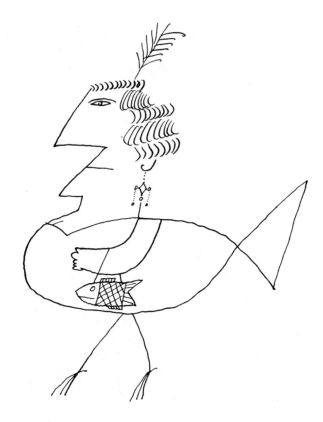

in the sort of dreams that accompany sexual excitement. Too pre-occupied as we are with ordinary shortcomings and bodily afflictions to muse about our wingless state, the disability nevertheless gnaws, unknown to us, at our entrails. Occasionally, release from our earthly bonds is granted in sleep when we are propelled into bird-like flight.

Only in our dreams do we achieve an angel's uplift and airy grace. Then, gravity drops off like an ugly scab, and we find that we can levitate or soar like a lark. Dreaming, we are able to outleap any ballet dancer; to perform high jumps in slow motion; to float per-pendicularly or horizontally above the ground, or to kneel in mid-air. Significantly, these nocturnal excursions are not undertaken in an immaterial, ghostlike state but in the full awareness of our body, indeed, of its dress. From firsthand accounts we learn that air turbu-lences do not dismay the dreamer; however, in conformity with the morals of the day, he does not forget the rudiments of decency. Our

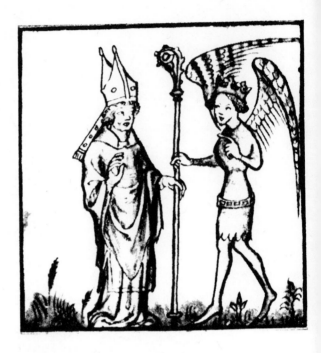

Miniskirted Angel. Le Roman de la Rose. *Manuscript, c. 1380. (Courtesy, The Trustees of the Pierpont Morgan Library)*

260

great-grandmothers, paragons of modesty that they were, preserved decorousness while soloing at giddy heights; "I attempt," one veteran flyer testified, "to drape my skirts chastely around my legs." Wings or no wings, flying dreams have been diagnosed as either the expression of erotic wishes, or an atavistic hangover from the time when some of our arboreal ancestors leaped from branch to branch among the trees. On the authority of such disparate thinkers as Plato and Freud, dreams are the workings of desire to satisfy itself in imagery when the higher faculties no longer inhibit our passions.

Where does all this leave the angels? What is the connection between wings and sexuality?

From time immemorial, rustling wings have denoted an amorous disposition and a penchant for amorous intrigue. Psyche, of Amor & Psyche, the personification of the human soul, was generally represented as a winged maiden in accordance with the old notion of the soul as a bird or insect. Or, for another example, Hermes, alias Mercury, "conductor of dreams," consort of Pan and the nymphs, whose image is sometimes reduced in artistic shorthand to a phallus, wears detachable wings, fastened to his sandals. Is one correct in assuming that these little wings are the badge of libertinism? It would seem so; the archetype of matchmakers, Greek *erotes*, who became naturalized in the old Rome as *amores* and *cupidines*, are a winged breed. On the whole, cupids are hard to distinguish from baby angels.

Whichever way one looks at them, wings represent far more than a flying apparatus. They are both metaphor—we speak of the wings of sleep, the wings of death—and a decorative appendage. As the latter they play a considerable role in the courtship of birds: The male bird spreads his wings before the female, much as a woman flaunts her décolletage at man. Wings also adorn a number of symbolic, pre-angelesque creatures. The aforementioned sphinxes, griffins, and assorted plumed animal figures of Egypt and Assyria that stood sentry at palace and temple doors, were so necessary to human imagination that later they reappeared in Greek and Roman art. (Their biblical counterpart is the angel who barred the way to the tree of life in Paradise.) Clearly, angels are the only heavenly bodies in the Christian-Jewish-Islamic pantheon that stand comparison with the winged divinities of heathen worlds.

Another accessory relegated to myth and religion is the halo, shining proof of man's perfectibility. It was already old hat, so to speak, long before being conferred upon the Christian godhead and the legions of saints. In classical times it had been standard equipment of, among others, the sun god Helios, the moon goddess Selene, and Eos, the rosy dawn. Also Buddha's low-slung halo—it is more in the nature of a peignoir rather than a wide brim—by far antedates the canonical nimbus. Indeed, not until the fifth century A.D. did Christianity claim the heathen halo its own, and even then it appeared only in the dimly lit mural paintings of catacombs. At first the exclusive attribute of Christ, in time it became a fixture of the mother of God, the angels, saints, and apostles, as well as of some Old Testament non-canonized figures.

The halo's effect on the face it frames goes far beyond the flattery of ordinary headgear such as a hat, a crown, or a wig. Apart from proclaiming the wearer's permanent state of grace, it overflows with radiance, sending gusts of holiness down his shoulders. It lends an extra air of confidence to the saints who adorn a predella, looking like dolls in a toy shop. A halo may be chipped, its gilt faded or dulled, cured by the smoke of altar candles, yet its fit is always impeccable. Martyrs writhing in flames, being halved or quartered, drowned or nailed to a cross, are never caught with their haloes dangling or askew. Although a saintly head may have been severed by the executioner's ax, the halo clings to it in defiance of all natural laws.

Occasionally, emperors hovering on the brink of godliness, or other mortals of exalted station, did not hesitate to have a halo incorporated into their portraits. Artists, poorly acquainted with protocol, had no scruples to confer it on such important, albeit

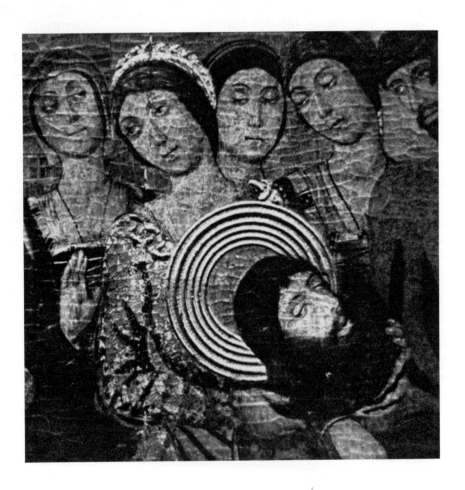

The beheaded St. John the Baptist with his halo in place. Detail. Catalan School.

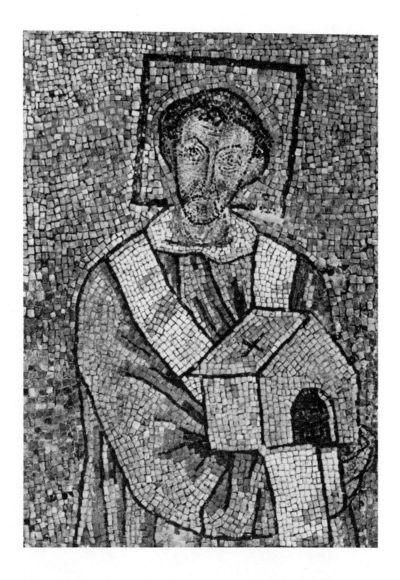

unholy persons as Herod or that notorious sinner, Theodora. But then, the halo as symbol of power and sovereignty was nothing new; it has precedents in the Orient. Indian kings of the first and the following centuries were portrayed haloed. So was Alexander the Great. Nero became the first Roman to usurp the holy disk, and at least one pope, John VII, while still alive, had himself immemorialized with a square halo in a mosaic at St. Peter's Basilica. (Christian iconography also comprises a few haloed animals. By taking a hint from the Greeks' halation of the mythical

Phoenix—the everlasting bird later turns up also in Christian art—
the Church glorified the lamb of Christ and the dove of the Holy
Spirit.)

Millinery fashions being what they are it was perhaps inevitable
that some artists tried to improve on the circular halo. The resulting
variations, unknown in Puritan countries with their dearth of saints,
are worth noting because they reveal rare instances of the artist's
unconcern with conventional attire. The square halo flourished
from the eighth to the thirteenth century, a long stretch of time
for so capricious a fashion. By no means the brainchild of a mad
hatter, it served graphically to distinguish the living from the dead
among the portrayed. It must not be confused with the rectangular

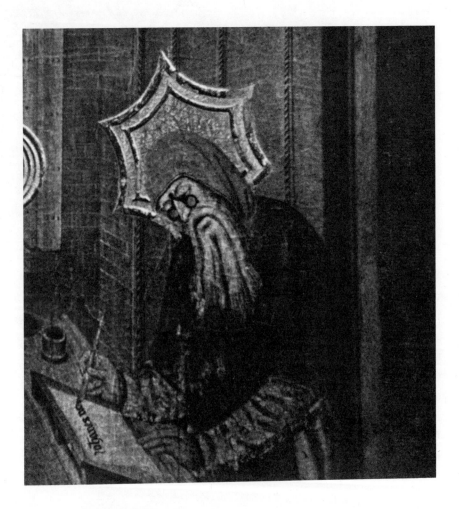

Polygonal, scalloped halo. Catalan School.

halo which—around the year 1000—became a common accessory of mundane dignitaries and patrons of art.

After successfully squaring the circle, painters invented ever more advanced models, such as halos of triangular and polygonal shape. Nor did these exhaust the repertory; ancient coins and bas-reliefs record a sampling of halos in the form of starry crowns, snow crystals, arrows of light—issuing, as it were, from the occiput—and concentric circles that later were reduced to a simple hoop.

The halo's coloration was anything but stereotyped. Before the Church settled for a sort of gold standard, artists favored cool shades. Blue and green halos prevail in early Christian murals.

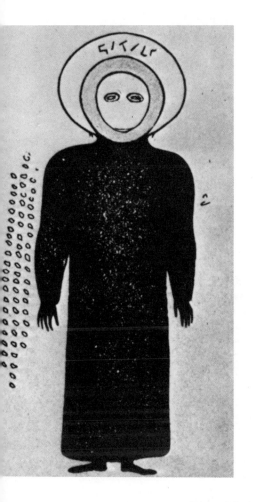 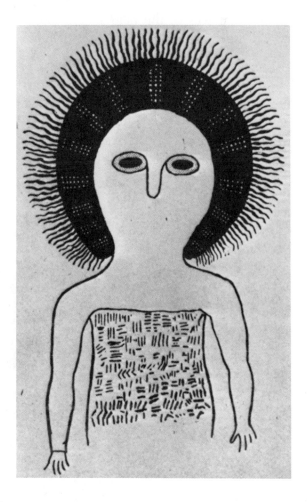

Haloed figures from a cave painting by aboriginal Australians.
Journal of the Royal Anthropological Institute of Great Britain.

Pale yellow, or more precisely a wheat color bordered by white and black, was the thing to wear from the fifth to the ninth century. In one instance the hand of God is shown surrounded by a blue-red-blue aureole but eventually egg yellow became the norm. Means permitting, the holy disk was gold-plated, often in fancy patterns, or inlaid with a cross and the saint's initials.

The halo's origin is obscure. Some art historians have traced it to a misunderstanding. According to their prosaic way of thinking, the symbol of godliness and holiness is derived from a most primitive contraption, the metal disk which the Greeks used to place at the top of statues to protect them from being defiled by bird droppings. It is an unattractive theory and does not account for the halo's vertical position, for obviously the halo is not so much a headcovering as a foil. Less banal though equally questionable is the theory that sees in the halo an offshoot from the parasol. The sunshade was indeed the traditional attribute of Assyrian and Persian royalty as well as the crowning feature of India's Buddhist stupas. But its transition to the halo with its ninety-degree turnabout remains unexplained.

There is poetic justice in the fact that the halo cannot be adapted to apparel. Neither can it be transposed into the third dimension; it simply defies materialization, with the exception of Buddha's golden mantle. Sculptors have grappled in vain with the problem

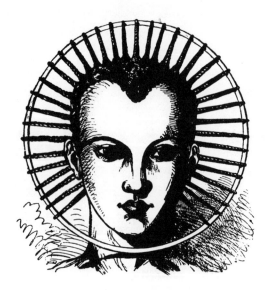

This African hairdo—thirty-seven pigtails attached to a hoop—resembles, as Livingstone observed, "the glory round the head of the Virgin."
From Missionary Travels *by David Livingstone.*

of how to launch the halo into space and make it stay there. The results are unconvincing. The necessity of attaching it to the head by means of a metal rod robs it of its wonderousness; the upshot is a saucepan effect. Stylized in stone it becomes absurd, a petrified mortarboard.

Only slightly less dazzling a breed than angels are heroes. The word hero has to be understood not as the current euphemism so readily applied to soldiers and football stars but in its original meaning: a man whose superhuman qualities and achievements make him eligible for the company of the immortals. By vigorously stretching the point, one might also include the canonized statesman. Purged of trivialities, he emerges a minor godhead. His core of morality having been laid bare, his career tidied up, his philanderings forgotten, he becomes the common property of generations of mythmakers. A grateful nation's tribute to him are memorial days and historical plays in which he comes to life for the duration of the performance. But whenever the need is felt for a more tangible, permanent homage—such as an effigy in bronze or stone—a problem arises for which no etiquette book has an answer.

The artist whose task it is to portray the great man in full figure is not so much in doubt whether to show him standing, seated, or lying down as to decide what he ought to wear in perpetuity. (The question of an equestrian monument is not likely to come up; no contemporary artist would want to invite comparison with Donatello or Verrocchio.) Whether the national hero has been dead for generations or has just recently passed away, the sculptor has to find means for doing him sartorial justice. Unlike the painter he simply cannot slur over his external appearance. Three possibilities are open to him: He can show the man in that singularly neutral state, the nude or semi-nude. Although this expedient worked well at other times and in other countries, we are not in sympathy with such frivolity. An equally unhappy solution is to dress him in the sort of clothes he wore during his lifetime. If he lived to an old age, they may comprise the wardrobe of two or three generations: knee breeches and silk stockings or baggy trousers; a curly wig, a plumed hat, a top hat, a walking stick, and all the excess baggage of human dignity. Hence the artist must decide whether he wants

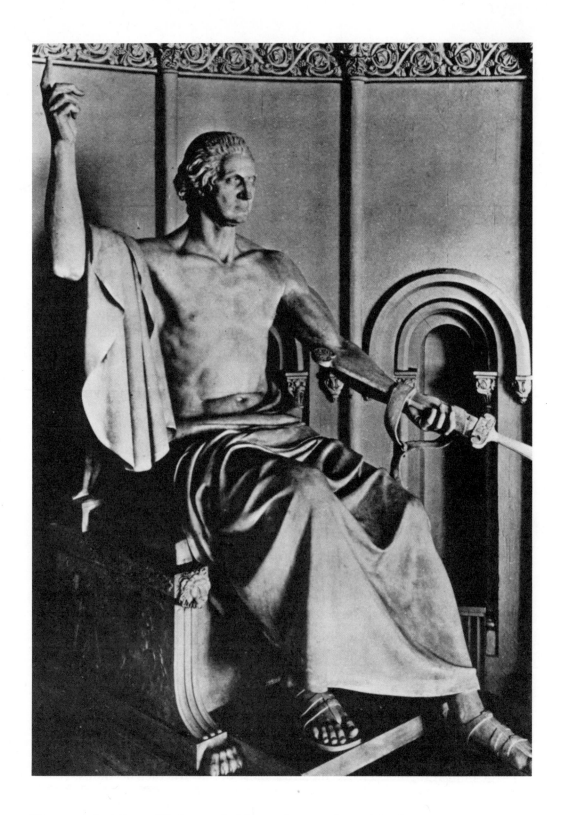

The semi-naked George Washington by Horatio Greenough scandalized a nation jealously guarding its moral purity. Instead of, as intended, adorning one of the capital's hallowed places, it languishes in a state institution. (Courtesy, Smithsonian Institution)

to stress quaintness—the time lag of provincialism—or show his hero as a cosmopolitan dandy. Alas, all tailors' fashions carry the germ of future ridicule so that sculptors run the risk of ending up with a monumental scarecrow rather than a monument. Moreover, the thought of translating a fashion plate, complete with lapels, buttons and pockets, perky bow and trouser crease, into metal or stone is anathema to them.

The third approach, a favorite though by no means infallible one, is to withdraw into anachronism. For some inexplicable reason, emperors' clothes of the classical variety seem best to satisfy our unsure taste. They have served in centuries past as an all-purpose costume for statues and murals, and for want of a better solution will probably serve for centuries to come. Horatio Greenough—to take up the case of an American artist—in portraying the Father of the Country adopted a middle course between the first and last alternatives. His Washington avoids the pitfalls of both the nude and full dress. The torso is timelessly naked while, from the navel down, the garment—if one can call it that—is noncommittally antiquarian. For breeches and boots has been substituted a shroud that would drop to the floor should Washington, in imitation of the Commendatore in *Don Giovanni*, want to get up to crush the hand of any living President. On his feet he sports a pair of sandals, something he surely would have refused to wear even for a masked ball. There can be little doubt that, had he ever dared to show himself in the street in this or a similar outlandish outfit, his career would have come to a sudden end. If anything, Washington's locker-room négligé expresses a sculptor's allergy to modern apparel.

As was to be expected, this large-scale marble monument, the first ever carved by a native artist, aroused the wrath of a prurient nation; "purblind squeemishness," complained Greenough, "awoke with a roar at the colossal nakedness of Washington's manly breast."[123] As a consequence, the statue, intended to be placed beneath the vaulted arch of the Capitol, was relegated to the park grounds where it languished half hidden by shrubbery. Eventually, the ostracized work of art was granted asylum at Washington's Smithsonian Institution. Two recent competitions for monuments honoring Franklin D. Roosevelt and John F. Kennedy respectively, ended inconclusively. The prize-winning artists, perhaps in order to fend off the very insinuation that they were willing to condone figurative sculpture in our time, presented a modified version of the currently fashionable type of outdoor art, those obstacle courses of cement and stone slabs commonly referred to as playground sculpture.

"Why this desire to dehumanize," asked Ortega y Gasset; "why this disgust at living forms? Why is it that the round and soft forms of living bodies are repulsive to the present-day artist?"[124] It remains for the anthropologist to supply the answer why so few modern artists stoop to representing the human form, nude or clothed. Painters and sculptors alike scorn clothes as a pictorial subject. At best they treat them in a summary way, as a tedious convention rather than a splendid foil. Ruskin could still rhapsodize on clothes in art without exposing himself to ridicule because in his time they were considered a legitimate pictorial subject, in no way inferior to a nude or a landscape. "I feel confident in your general admiration," he told a lecture audience apropos some Reynolds portraits, "that the charm of all these pictures is in a great degree dependent on toilettes; that the fond and graceful flatteries of each master do in no small measure consist in his management of frillings and trimmings, cuffs and collarettes; and on beautiful flingings and fastenings of investiture . . . "[125] Today, an artist's eye rarely focuses on dress, and then mainly on its absurdities. Only the satirist and social critic among artists finds dress a source of stimulation.

Saul Steinberg, the foremost contemporary chronicler of the human comedy, has what amounts to a vested interest in sartorial fantasy. Yet he never caricatures the day's fashions; in fact, he invariably adds to his work an ever so faint anachronistic touch, just enough to lift it above mere actuality. When he arrived on the American scene, that icon of piercing purity and grandest datable monument to native womanhood, the Gibson Girl, had long been melted down in the nation's caldron and recast in a more profane vein. "It struck me," he recalls, "that women were dressed and painted like prostitutes. I understood this later: in America, there is no tradition of professional prostitution as in Europe, where

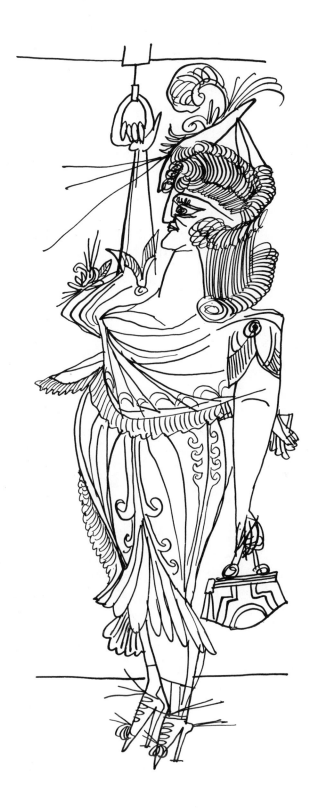

Drawing by Saul Steinberg. From The Catalogue. *Copyright © 1945.*

honest women have to dress like honest women, and a sexy outfit denotes a profession."

Today, Steinberg is able to pool thirty years' observation into a single shorthand drawing. He likes to show women with their sails unfurled, so to speak, or covered with a parasitic flora of symbols. The corrosive quality of their clothes is surpassed only by that of their footwear; "the shoes themselves," he points out, "are aggressive."[126] Although he can get as much entranced with the minutiae of dress as any old master, his first concern is not with the trappings but with the human being underneath them. This accounts no doubt for the fact that the clothes he depicts with so much gusto often look more like emanations of their wearer than products of the garment industry.

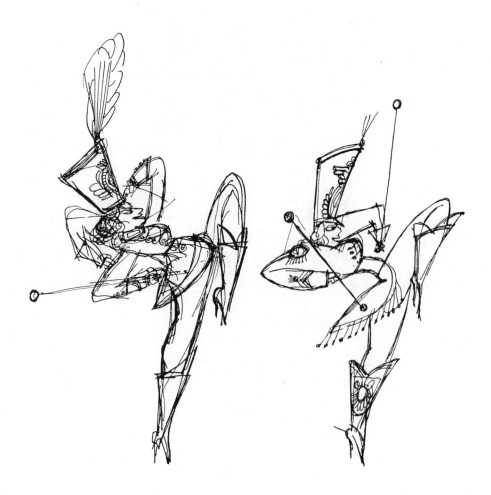

"Drum majorettes," drawing by Saul Steinberg.
From The Passport. *Copyright © 1954.*

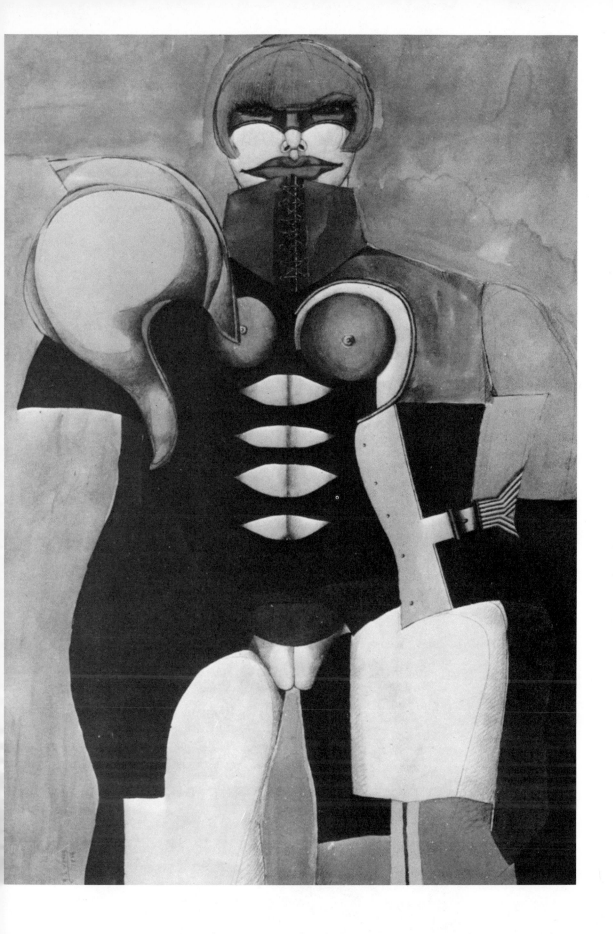

Some of the more sinister aspects of form-fitting apparel are captured in Nancy Grossman's work. Below: "Head in wood and leather. (Courtesy, Cordier and Ekstrom, New York). Opposite: "Figure," drawing, 1970. (Courtesy, Dieter Brusberg)

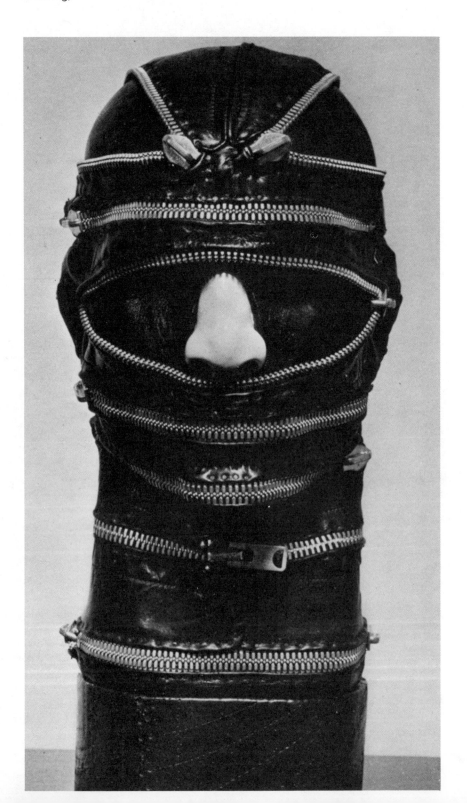

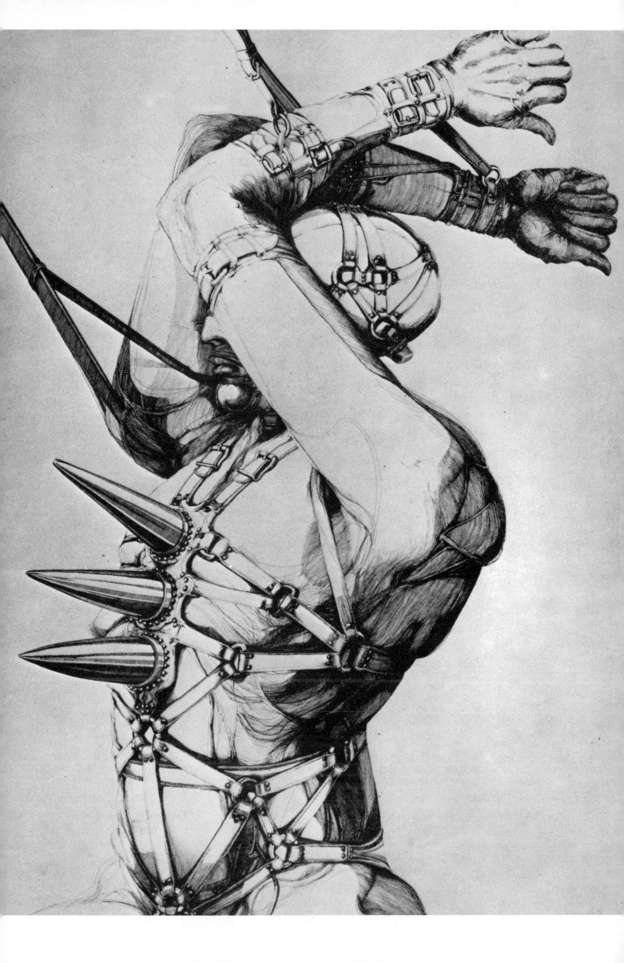

Christo, whose packaged woman we encountered on page 229, dilates upon the cruelty rather than the elegance of clothes. His way with them is offhand, albeit magisterial. A wedding gown he composed for the 1966 city-wide Arts Festival in Philadelphia also illustrates his flair for an eerie sort of grandeur. The bridal train consisted of an enormous package—perhaps the weightiest metaphor on record—confectioned from four hundred square feet of white satin. It was pulled by a young woman harnessed to two hundred feet of silk rope. Christo, one of the more baffling members of the new vanguard, here is at his enigmatic best. In dealing with the farcical and ludicrous he expends unlimited poetic license and although most of his work is sober to the point of asceticism, it easily takes its place with the aching riddles of the Sphinx. Some of his critics have perceived a whiff of the morgue, a vague air of

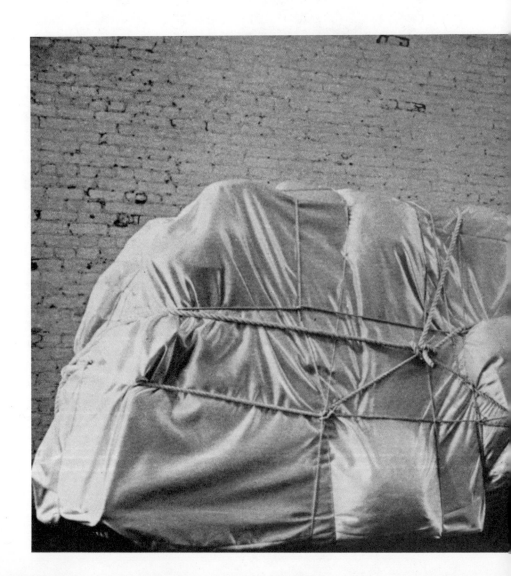

crime about his smaller sculptures, and compared them to exhibits of judiciary evidence. Others have likened the spell exuded by his objects to that of ventriloquism, sword swallowing, and acts of mystification in general. And in a sense he is truly a purveyor of daytime nightmares.

What does the bridal charade stand for? Does the woman suggest the original slave, man's beast of burden dragging her dowry or is she simply the artist's muse parading one of his prize packages? Or, given the facts that Christo was born less than one hundred miles from Greece and enjoyed a European classical education, are we presented with a take-off on the Panathenaic Procession where Athenian maidens carried the new robes through the streets to the Acropolis to clothe the goddess' image? Come to think of it, Christo's wrappings *are* Greek drapery transposed into contemporary idiom.

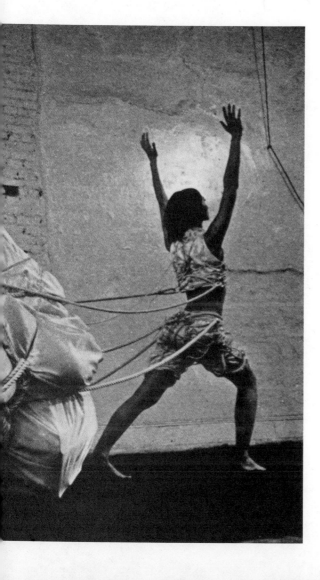

"Bridal gown," by Christo. 1967.

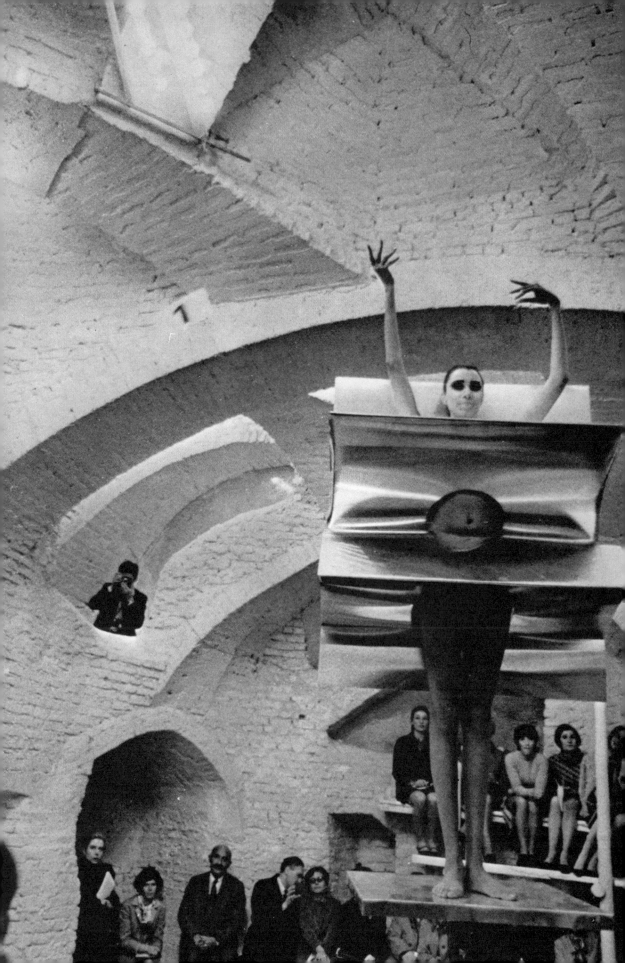

On the assumption that a parable on clothes is dull to write about but entertaining enough to be acted out, William Klein, the American painter, photographer, and film maker, who lives and works in Paris, decided to indulge his prodigious talent for persiflage by staging a mock fashion show. Having spent many years as a student of the *haute couture*'s seasonal myths, he was singularly equipped to deal with its aesthestic maunderings. The vehicle that served to make his point was *Qui Êtes-Vous Polly Maggoo?* a film about an American fashion magazine cover girl's tribulations and rise to glory.

Films have a tendency to fade as fast as flowers taken from a florist's refrigerator, and none more so than those that dispense social comment. To sustain the pungency of his satire within a satire, Klein had to find clothes that not only would not be outdated by the time the film was released but would seem sufficiently grotesque in years to come. Thus, in terms of clothes design, the task he set himself was all but impracticable. "To ask Courrèges—who was then [in 1965] the whiz kid of the moment—or other dress designers was useless," explained Klein, "since by definition their ideas are instantly obsolete. So I thought of doing something completely absurd as well as absolutely unwearable." Wood, stone, steel, though preposterous enough as dress materials, present all sorts of difficulties to tailoring. Besides, they might turn out to be unflattering to the wearer, and nothing could be more intolerable to the artist. However frenetic his farce, on no account would he forsake Gallic elegance. The solution that presented itself were aluminum dresses, adapted from the celebrated musical instruments of François and Bernard Baschet.

Piling irony on sarcasm, Klein invited the press and the *real* world of fashion to play the part of the public in the film's fashion show. In a monastic setting reminiscent of the first Christians' secret meeting places, he deposited his works of art on a wave of admiration. The hallucinatory parade of armor-plated women put the most acidulous critics *hors de combat*; "you are more than a creator, you are a galvanizer," punned one man of letters. Thus, what had been intended as mockery, dissolved in an atmosphere of general euphoria. To Klein's dismay—mixed, to be sure, with

The 1966 vogue in metal clothes was triggered by an artist's jest, the fashion show in William Klein's satirical film "Qui Êtes-Vous Polly Maggoo?"

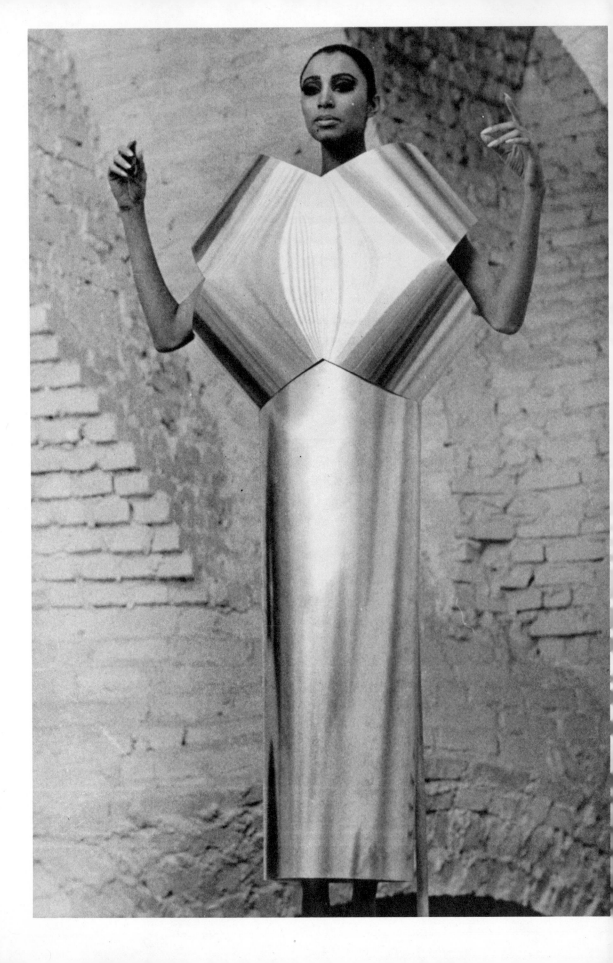

glee—the gowns were applauded as "tomorrow's fashion." Evidently, fashionable dress, and the hokum that surrounds it, are impervious to parody.

As in every edifying fable, the hero's defeat eventually turned into a triumph. The most potent piece of news that emerged from the Paris collections in the summer of 1966 were metal dresses and metal moulages. "Polly" came out in October, and by Christmas all the stores had tin-, silver-, and gold-foil garments in their windows.

This glorious, sonorous garment, a show stopper in Klein's film "Polly," was adapted by François and Bernard Baschet from their celebrated musical instruments.

Text references

1. Jakob Ludwig Karl Grimm, *Household Tales*. London, 1884, p. 98.
2. Jakob Ludwig Karl Grimm, *German Household Tales*. Boston and New York, 1897, p. viii.
3. Georges Auguste Morache, *Pékin et ses habitants*. Paris, 1869, p. 97.
4. *The Works of Jacob Behmen* (Boehme). London, 1772, vol. III, chap. 18, p. 73.
5. Ibid., p. 75.
6. Ibid., p. 73.
7. Charles Chauncey, *Five Dissertations on the Scriptures Account of the Fall*, etc. London, 1785, p. 85.
8. Micha Joseph Berdyczewski, *Die Sagen der Juden*. Frankfurt, 1913–27.
9. Alfred Ernest Crawley, *Dress, Drinks, and Drums*. London, 1931, p. 11.
10. Jean Baptiste Tavernier, *Orientalische Reiss-Beschreibung*. Genff, 1681, 4. Buch, 12. Capitel, p. 197.
11. Johann Wilhelm Helfer, *Reisen in Vorderasien*. Vienna, 1859, vol. II, p. 12.
12. Edward Westermarck, *The History of Human Marriage*. New York, 1922, vol. I, p. 535.
13. "Unveiled Women Stir Syrian Riot" (*New York World Telegram*, May 7, 1945).
14. John McMaster, *A History of the People of the United States*. New York, 1910, vol. 6, p. 96.
15. John Bulwer, *Anthropometamorphosis*. London, 1653, p. 502.
16. Jacques Boileau, *A just and seasonable Reprehension of naked Breasts*, etc. London, 1678, p. 16.
17. "Lindsay Assails Topless Attire" (*The New York Times*, January 14, 1967).
18. Céline Renooz, *Psychologie Comparée de l'Homme et da la Femme*. Passy-Paris, 1897, p. 85.
19. *Catalogue of prints and drawings in the British Museum*. Division I, Satires, vol. III, pt. I, p. 744.

20. Erasmus Darwin, *Zoönomia*. Dublin, 1800, vol. I, p. 174.
21. Havelock Ellis, *Studies in the Psychology of Sex*. New York, 1942, vol. IV, p. 113.
22. Marie d'Aulnoy, *La cour et la ville de Madrid*. Paris, 1874, vol. 1, p. 271.
23. Louis de Rouvray, *Mémoires*. Paris, 1853–58, vol. 18, p. 370.
24. d'Aulnoy, op. cit., vol. I, p. 180.
25. *Funk and Wagnalls Standard Dictionary of Folklore, Mythology and Legend*. New York, 1949–50, p. 1008.
26. Jacob Nacht, *Symbolism of the Shoe with special References to Jewish Sources*. London, 1915, p. 11.
27. McMaster, op. cit., vol. 6, p. 96.
28. F. Somerville (*Journal of the Anthropological Institute*, London, 1894, p. 368).
29. Bulwer, op. cit., p. 348.
30. "Men and their Looks" (*Vogue*, New York, Nov. 15, 1966).
31. John Carl Flügel, *The Psychology of Clothes*. London, 1930, p. 193.
32. James Augustus St. John, *Oriental Album*. London, 1851, p. 27.
33. Charles Nicolas Sigisbert Sonnini de Manoncourt, *Voyage dans le Haute et Basse Egypte*. Paris, 1779, vol. I, p. 289.
34. Dunlap Knight, *Personal Beauty and Racial Betterment*. St. Louis, 1920, p. 28.
35. William Shakespeare, *Othello*, Act I, Sc. 3.
36. Bulwer, op. cit., p. 502.
37. Pliny the Elder, *Natural History*. London, 1942, Book VII, I. 5–8, p. 521.
38. Eckart von Sydow, "Primitive Kunst und Psychoanalyse" (*Imago-Bücher*, Leipzig, 1927, Band 10, p. 153).
39. Charles Darwin, *The Descent of Man*. New York, n.d., p. 890.
40. James Hastings, *Encyclopaedia of Religion and Ethic*. New York, 1951, p. 898.
41. *Encyclopedia Americana*. New York, 1957, vol. 22, p. 22.
42. L. W. G. Malcolm, "Note on the Seclusion of Girls among the Efik at Old Calabar" (*Man*, London, 1925, p. 113).
43. Darwin, op. cit., p. 886.
44. Hermann Heinrich Ploss, *Woman, an historical, gynaecological and anthropological compendium*. London, 1935, vol. I, p. 447.
45. Peter Simon Pallas, *Travels through the Southern Provinces of the Russian Empire in the Years 1793–94*. London, 1812, p. 398.
46. Thorstein Veblen, *The Theory of the Leisure Class*. New York, 1911, p. 172.
47. Ellis, op. cit., vol. II, part 1, p. 172.
48. "Modern English Dandy" (*Current Literature*, New York, 1903, vol. 34, p. 228).
49. Simon J. Wikler and Thomas Hale, "Gross Non-painful Foot Defects" (*Military Medicine*, October 1965, vol. 130, no. 10).
50. Adolfo Dembo and J. Imbelloni, "Deformaciones" (*Humanior*, Buenos Aires, 1938, seccion A, tome 3, p. 3).
51. Bernard Rudofsky, *The Kimono Mind*. New York, 1964, p. 50.
52. Bulwer, op. cit., p. 379.
53. Raphael Patai, *Sex and Family in the Bible and the Middle East*. New York, 1959, p. 201.
54. Ellis, op. cit., vol. II, part 3, p. 172.

55. Arthur Schopenhauer, *Parerga und Paralipomena*. Berlin, 1851, vol. II, p. 482.
56. Ibid., vol. I, p. 190.
57. Bulwer, op. cit., p. 46.
58. "Kheel Splits Hair in Backing Transit Employee on Vandyke" (*The New York Times*, April 15, 1965).
59. Bronislaw Malinowski, *The Sexual Life of Savages in North-Western Melanesia*. London, 1929, p. 335.
60. Darwin, op. cit., p. 852.
61. Ibid., p. 882.
62. Ibid.
63. L. Higgin, *Art as applied to dress*. London, 1885, p. 45.
64. "Shaw's Ideas on Garb" (*Harper's Weekly*, April 1, 1905, vol. 49, p. 457).
65. John Evelyn, *Tyrannus or The Mode*. Oxford, 1951, p. 25.
66. Henry Holiday, "How Men Dress—The Tubular System" (*English Illustrated Magazine*, London, September 1893, no. 120, p. 909).
67. Flügel, op. cit., p. 35.
68. Lady F. W. Haberton, "Symposium on Dress" (*Arena*, New York, 1892, vol. 6, p. 622).
69. Gordon Rattray Taylor, *Sex in History*. New York, 1954, p. 82.
70. Helena Maria Webber in Frances E. Russell, "A Brief Survey of the American Dress Reform Movement of the Past" (*Arena*, New York, 1892, vol. 6, p. 491).
71. Edmund Russell, "Symposium on Women's Dress" (*Arena*, New York, 1892, vol. 6, p. 491).
72. Elizabeth Stuart Phelps in Frances E. Russell, "A Brief Survey of the American Dress Reform Movement of the Past" (*Arena*, New York, 1892, vol. 6, p. 333).
73. Ibid., p. 326.
74. Maria M. Jones, *Woman's Dress: Its Moral and Physical Relations*. New York, 1864, p. 22.
75. Ibid., p. 17.
76. Mary E. Tillotson, *History ov the first thirty-five years ov the science costume movement in the United States*. Vineland, N.J., 1885, p. 17.
77. Grace Greenwood in "Symposium on Women's Dress" (*Arena*, New York, 1892, vol. 6, p. 632).
78. Lato (pseud.), *So-called Skirts*. London, 1906, p. 62.
79. J. J. Jenny (*Ciba Symposia*, Summit, N.J., December 1944, p. 1975).
80. Gustav Jäger, *A Treatise on Health Culture*. New York, 1886, p. 37.
81. Ibid., p. 87.
82. Gustav Jäger, *Selections from Essays on Health Culture*. New York, 1891, p. 73.
83. Ibid., p. 138.
84. Ibid., p. 139.
85. Paul Gentizon, "La querelle des coiffures; du turban au chapeau par le fez" (*Mercure de France*, Paris, November 1, 1927, p. 317).
86. Lord Stanmore, Governor of Fiji, quoted in Havelock Ellis, *Studies in the Psychology of Sex*. New York, 1942, vol. IV, p. 100.
87. Robert Burton, *Anatomy of Melancholy*. Oxford, 1624, part III, sec. 2, sub-sec. 3, p. 374.

88. Mario Praz, *The Romantic Agony*. London, 1933, p. 197.

89. Gérard de Nerval, *Aurélia*. Paris, 1965, p. 4.

90. *Journal de Eugène Delacroix*. Paris, 1932, vol. I, p. 152.

91. Mary Wortley Montagu, *Letters of the Right Honourable Lady M-y W-y M-u Written during her Travels in Europe, Asia and Africa*, etc. Aix, 1796, p. 111.

92. Ibid., p. 120.

93. William James, *The Principles of Psychology*. New York, 1890, vol. II, p. 435.

94. Albert Moll, *Sexual Life of the Child*. New York, 1923, p. 91.

95. John Ryan, *Prostitution in London*. London, 1839, p. 382.

96. Ellis, op. cit., vol. I, part 2, p. 154.

97. J. Sadger, "Psychoanalyse eines Autoerotikers" (*Jahrbuch für psychoanalytische Forschungen*. Leipzig, 1913, Bd. 5, p. 502).

98. Hilaire Hiler, *Costumes and Ideologies*. New York, 1939, p. xvii.

99. *Encyclopaedia Biblica*. New York, 1899, vol. I, p. 170.

100. Isaiah 3, 16–20.

101. Georg August Schweinfurth, *The Heart of Africa*. New York, 1874, vol. I, p. 153.

102. *Journal of the Anthropological Society of Bombay*, vol. III, p. 370.

103. David Livingstone, *Missionary Travels*, etc. London, 1857, p. 276.

104. "A Modest Emperor" (*The New York Times*, December 28, 1967).

105. Isabel Burton, *The Inner Life of Syria, Palestine, and the Holy Land*. London, 1875, vol. II, p. 1.

106. Thomas Coryat, *Coryat's Crudities*. Glasgow and New York, 1905, vol. I, p. 400.

107. Pompeo Gherardo Molmenti, *La storia di Venezia nella vita privata*. Bergamo, 1908–11, vol. I, p. 282.

108. Rudofsky, op. cit., p. 49.

109. Ellis, op. cit., vol. I, part 2, p. 158.

110. Ibid., vol. III, part 1, p. 106.

111. *Indiae Orientalis*. Francoforti, 1612, pars nona, p. 21.

112. Benjamin Frederik Matthes, *Bijdragen tot de Ethnologia van Zuider-Celebes*. Amsterdam, 1875, p. 35.

113. Fritz Grabowsky, "Die 'Orang bukit' oder Bergmenschen von Mindai in Ost-Borneo" (*Das Ausland*, München, 1885, VIII, p. 785).

114. Matthes, op. cit., p. 35.

115. William Marsden, *The History of Sumatra*. London, 1784, p. 44.

116. Heinrich Sundermann, *Die Insel Nias*. Berlin, 1884, p. 443.

117. James Sibree, *Madagascar and its People*. London, 1870, p. 193.

118. Richard Irving Dodge, *Our Wild Indians*. Hartford, 1890, p. 196.

119. Granville Stanley Hall, *Adolescence*. New York, 1922, vol. II, p. 113.

120. *The Art Criticism of John Ruskin*. New York, 1964, p. 262.

121. George Clayton, *Angelology*. New York, 1851, p. 134.

122. Ovid, *Ars amatoria* (Loeb). Cambridge, 1962, vol. II, p. 71.

123. Horatio Greenough, *Aesthetics at Washington*. Washington, 1851, p. 6.

124. José Ortega y Gasset, *The Dehumanization of Art*. New York, 1956, p. 39.

125. Ruskin, op. cit., p. 336.

126. Jean vanden Heuvel, "Steinberg" (*Life*, Chicago, December 10, 1965, p. 64).

Index

Photographers' credits

Alinari 22, 129, 249, 253, 263; Ferdinand Boesch 229; Henry Clarke 201; Geoffrey Clements 272, 273, 275; Eliot Elisofon 95, 138; Hans Martin von Erffa 64; William Klein 278, 280; Ugo Mulas 38; Jack Nisberg 217; Arthur Penn 36, 61, 68; Bernard Rudofsky 20, 24, 45, 56, 81, 83, 88, 114, 135, 150, 159, 192, 215, 235, 257, 262, 264; Franco Rubartelli 136; Shunk-Kender 276; Bert Stern 213, 219; Soichi Sunami 122, 123; Barbara Sutro 46, 188; Charles Wilp 198.